Natural Birth

A Holistic Guide to Pregnancy, Childbirth and Breastfeeding

Kristina Turner

Floris Books

*Woman gets soul with child. Not necessary
have child, necessary readiness for child.*

G.I. Gurdjieff

First published by Floris Books 2010

© 2010 Kristina Turner
Illustrations by Adam Turner and Bobby Sephton

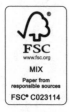

British Library CIP Data available
ISBN 978-086315-763-9
Printed in Great Britain
by Page Bros (Norwich) Ltd

Contents

Opening your Mind to a
Different View of Childbirth

Most of us would say that we want a quick and painless birth and, indeed, a quick and painless death. We are seeking to avoid rather than to transform.

We can choose to consider ourselves the victims of whatever happens to us in life, in which case we are forever at the mercy of chance events, at the mercy of accidents. We can also choose to transform what happens to us by opting for the most practical interpretation of events, practical being that interpretation which most benefits our development and inner state.

Let us say, for example, that your car breaks down, leaving you late for a meeting. You can curse your bad luck, allow yourself to become overwhelmed by stress and irritation and arrive late at your meeting. Or you can strive to accept the breakdown as the best course of events: it may have prevented you from being involved in an accident which would have been the result of continuing to travel at high speed along the motorway — and arrive late at your meeting. In either case, the result is the same: you are late for your meeting. What is different, however, is your inner state.

In the former, you are a victim of circumstance and allow yourself to rage against this injustice, creating a negative state of mind. In the latter, you exercise your intelligence and ability to *transform* a chance accident into a positive inner state. This does not mean that we should unthinkingly try to put a positive spin on everything that happens in life, exclaiming after we have lost both hands in an accident, 'Hurrah, now I won't have to buy gloves any more!' The point is that we have more power over how we perceive reality than we think. And this means that we have a great deal more inner freedom than we think. Our outer freedom will always be limited by the chance events that shape our life, but we can learn to maintain our inner freedom.

The aim of existence is the transformation of substances. This will occur by itself, mechanically, through the transformation of food into movement, emotion and thought. It can also occur consciously, as a result of new knowledge and the subsequent change in how we behave, what we become. If we avoid difficulties in this life, we will avoid them in the next, and lose our opportunity to transform.

If we look at the Tibetan and Egyptian books describing what happens after death, they tell us that we are faced with the task of transformation. The descriptions of the deities vary according to culture or the principles they represent, but it is the aim of the living and the dead to develop and grow. The ladder of transformation leads all the way up to heaven. And if we allow ourselves to be governed by fear, our world becomes a small prison indeed.

If we look at birth with our ordinary mind, we could say that it is unbearably painful and massively exhausting. But our ordinary mind sees only dully, coldly and puts nothing in its proper context, where it is the rightful part of a much bigger whole. So it is with birthing.

What actually happened during my births could be observed from outside as a woman in increasing pain and labour, sweating, being sick, defecating and eventually pushing out a healthy baby. But there is a whole other side to the experience that I wish to address: the inner revelation which has the potential to affect us in a way so fundamental that our lives can be transformed by it. In comparison to this, the outer, bodily experiences wither.

By taking ourselves out of our normal state, in which we experience pain as discomfort, we can experience pain differently. It is possible to become temporarily free from the experiences of our physical bodies. The physical body does its work and responds to stimuli, but we are not as attached to it as usual. The experience then becomes one of overwhelming force, rather than pain. The effort is not really effort, because we are taken out of our usual state in which we wish to avoid effort. This is possible during birth and is one of the sacred initiation experiences attainable by women.

However, our abnormal living conditions mean that this no longer happens naturally, by itself. It requires preparation.

If we remain as we are, our real self covered in the stuff we have learned since childhood about what the body is and how to relate to it — if we believe that birth is painful, bloody and a necessary evil — then that is what it will be. We are the product of conditioning, upbringing and education, and our experiences will be accordingly: according to what we expect.

The potential birthing experience is truly great: a time out of time when a woman's body is allowed to become a vessel for forces infinitely greater than her, and the veil is lifted so that she may see, for a moment, the mysteries beyond time, death and birth. This is not something that we can just expect to happen by itself. What we can do is to prepare the body and psyche for experiencing something beyond the invisible assumptions through which our experience flows and finds its channels in the old well-worn grooves. After we have mapped what we are now and opened ourselves to possibilities beyond our social conditioning, perhaps, something new and infinitely greater may enter our world.

Three forces

In all the great religions, the number three is assigned special importance and is considered sacred. Here in the west, we are familiar with the idea of the Holy Trinity, and perhaps view it as an outmoded superstition. The significance of the number three runs deeper, however, and if we start to see the Holy Trinity as a symbolic representation of a cosmological law that has practical implications for our daily lives, it can begin to become useful to us.

Generally, we see only two: action and resistance. For example, the hedge needs cutting — I'm too busy. I tell my son to unload the dishwasher — he tells me it's his sister's turn. I want to get up early this Saturday so the whole day isn't wasted — my body keeps sleeping. These examples show a state of stand-off, where nothing can happen. These opposing forces are manifestations of the active and passive principles that are a fundamental part of the make-up of the cosmos. Most of the time we go through life stuck in 'like — don't like' mode. This makes life easier and is necessary to make life run smoothly. But if we become more aware, we can begin to experience the tension between the passive and active forces in our daily lives, and see how allowing dyads to govern all aspects of our lives can be limiting.

This is important in the context of childbirth because it will help you to see beyond the dichotomy of hospital birth versus home birth, authority versus victim, mainstream versus alternative and to think more for yourself, and in so doing take more responsibility for your experience.

Triads allow us to look at phenomena in terms of three forces. If we observe carefully, we will see that a phenomenon arises when a third force is introduced, which makes things happen. To continue the above example: the hedge needs cutting — I'm too busy — my neighbour comments on the tall hedge, which pushes me to cut it; I tell my son to unload the dishwasher — he tells me it's his sister's turn — I set up a rota, which prevents further arguments; I want to get up early this Saturday so the whole day isn't wasted — my body keeps sleeping — I set the alarm clock, which jolts my body out of resistance. The third force releases the tension of the two opposing forces and allows events and manifestations to take place by the meeting of active, passive and neutralizing forces.

The third force often seems to come from outside, and it is worth trying to observe this in our daily lives. Examples of triads I sometimes see are: the act of cooking (active), unprepared food (passive), hungry people (neutralizing); smoking (passive), wanting to quit (active), the expression in the child's eyes (neutralizing); like (active), don't like (passive), impartial (neutralizing): follow (passive), lead (active), dance (neutralizing).

On a deeper level, this is what the Holy Trinity speaks of. In Christianity it is symbolized by the triads of the Father, the Son and the Holy Ghost and Mary, Joseph and Jesus. To the ancient Egyptians, it was expressed as Amon, Mut and Khonsu. In Hinduism, we have the trinity of Brahma, Vishnu and Shiva.

One of the principal obstacles to understanding the significance of the three forces is our third-force blindness. We are taught from an early age to see things in terms of dyads, because it is easier and requires less of us as human beings: good — bad, right — wrong, pain — pleasure, black — white, us — them, friend — foe.

However, if we don't come down on one side or another in an argument or discussion, we maintain an open mind for longer and become more likely to think further, and so to be more empathetic. This implicitly means taking more responsibility for the situation we are in, because we don't categorize new experiences or ideas so quickly into good — bad, right — wrong and so on.

> The only real understanding that can ever be acquired depends upon a certain substance which can only be formed in a particular manner. This substance depends upon three factors: the presence of understandings of a like nature which become relatively positive and negative, and the new piece of knowledge which is the neutralizing force. The result of the three is a new understanding'.
> (A.R. Orage, from *The Oragean Version*, C. Daly King)

A warning

What kind of birth would you ideally want? Assume that you were free of the constraint of fear. All your 'buts' answered with, 'That will be taken care of, you need not worry.' If your answer is a natural birth, meaning as nature intended, without hospitals, machines or unnecessary intervention, then read on.

If you have given birth before you may have some doubts about natural childbirth, along the lines of, 'It's not actually that easy. It's all very well and good to come over all Earth Mother and talk about the joy of childbirth but the reality of it is a different matter. Well, how would you want your ideal birth to be?

Natural birth is not the only way. The ways to the truth are many, and each individual has his or her unique path to follow to the centre. Research the way you want to give birth and find your own way. Any way that works for you is valid and good. You will benefit from taking responsibility for your choices regardless of what they are.

1. An Introduction to Natural Birthing

What is natural birth?

Natural birth is a birth without interference. Emotional, psychological and physical support are not interference. Medical intervention in an emergency is not interference. Interference can be defined as something that is done to the birthing mother that she does not fully understand or even want, while being otherwise healthy. For example, using medical expertise which the mother is said not to possess in order to justify a surgical procedure or the administration of pharmaceuticals is interference.

A natural birth allows the instinctive processes to take their rightful course. The instinctive functions are much more sophisticated than the intellectual functions when it comes to running the chemical factory that we call the body. Instinctive functions operate at an unimaginable speed compared to our thinking faculty. The secretion of hormones, the circulation of the blood, the process of digestion, the repair of damaged tissue, the generation of bone marrow, the transmission of nerve impulses: all this goes on right under our own noses, in a fraction of the time it takes to even formulate this very sentence with our intellect. That is why induced birth can be so violent and painful. Compared to the delicate release and response system of our instinctive function, administering the hormone oxytocin artificially via a drip in the arm can only be crude and blunt, however finely calibrated by medical expertise.

Natural birth may involve pain, complications and death. Natural birth allows the forces of nature and God to work through a woman unencumbered by drugs, equipment and the restrictions of mechanical procedures. Natural birth can be, for the birthing woman, a point of connection with the reality that lies beyond time and matter.

Hospitals, machines and experts will be there if they are really needed. If anything goes 'wrong' during birth it is possible to go to hospital at any time. However, as those who have researched the field of natural childbirth and home birth will know, interference from doctors, machines and well-intentioned tinkering with a woman's finely-balanced systems can cause many of the complications that arise in hospital. This is examined in more detail in Chapter 9.

Giving birth naturally, through the vagina, allows the child to come into contact with microscopic particles of the mother's faeces, which contains bacteria that help the baby's immune system to develop properly. A link has been shown to exist between birth by caesarean section, where the baby does not come into contact with the mother's faeces, and the appearance of allergies in later life. Your baby is meant to come out through your vagina. The physiology of childbirth is no accident; it has been designed that way for a reason.

Another considerable benefit of natural childbirth is that during birth a woman's anatomy is shifted around slightly, which can make sex significantly more enjoyable after birth. When my first son's head passed through the opening of my vagina, all my tissues were pulled and stretched in such a way that I felt intense pleasure just as he emerged. This was surprising, almost shocking, as I had no idea that such a sensation could be associated with childbirth. After the further stretching of my perineum during the birth of my second child, my clitoris became optimally positioned for stimulation during intercourse. Part of me does not want to broadcast this to the world, but I will do it anyway; by including this possibility in the ether of our shared consciousness, it may become a reality for more women.

If you tape over the eyes of a newborn kitten, and remove the tape at eight weeks, the kitten will be blind for life. The potential function of sight did not receive any acknowledgment or stimulus, and so withered. It is possible to destroy something forever by pretending that it is not there, by never acknowledging that it is happening.

What is active birth?

Active birth is often used synonymously with natural birth. The woman is the instigator of events and the centre of the process of giving birth. Everyone present is focused on her and on supporting her in actively giving birth. In an active birth, a woman does not have things done to her. She has choice, authority, confidence. She receives support, assistance and advice. She is allowed to trust her body and the working of her instinctive function. She gives birth; her baby is not delivered.

What, then, is a good birth?

A good birth is what it is. This may sound obvious or simplistic, but take some time to think about it. To allow something to be what it is, without trying to change it, without trying to influence it, without trying to control it, without having expectations of it being something other than it actually is, is not commonplace. We are brought up to think that we can control our lives. If we work hard enough, we can make what we have decided upon happen.

I chose to study English at university. I chose to apply for a job in marketing. I chose to have a baby at 29. But did I really? I have completely forgotten about all the other possibilities that were available at the time. I also applied to study philosophy, but was not accepted. I also applied for a job in an art gallery but never got a reply. I had several miscarriages before the age of 29. A series of small accidents actually determined the events of my life. It *seems* as if I controlled events, got myself a degree in English, landed a job in marketing, had the children I always wanted. This apparent control over life events is an almost universally acknowledged truth in our culture.

If we take enough precautions, have enough screenings, eat the right food, keep fit, take the right supplements, we will almost certainly have a healthy baby and a healthy birth. This is the unspoken assumption. So how do we deal with the possibility of life bringing us grief, suffering and difficulties? Mostly, we pretend that they do not exist, which is also how we deal with death.

The possibility of birth also brings with it the possibility of death. Death is not something that we are taught how to deal with. Everyone who is struck by tragedy has to muddle through as best they can, perhaps with counselling or with the help of friends. We have lost most of the rituals that allow for the psychological transformation of death. We do not allocate any time for the passage, for the transition, both for the dead person and for those left behind in the world of matter.

Life will bring us difficulties, suffering and death. No one can avoid it, and pregnancy can end in the death of the child or the mother. We need to face this possibility too, and take responsibility for our attitude towards it. We tend to live our lives in such a way that if we cannot control the difficulties life brings, we expect someone else to do it for us, and we turn to doctors, counselling or medication to control life for us.

A good birth is not focused on avoiding difficulties. A good birth is one where the birthing mother is fully present, so that she may experience fully what is in *her* life. When she then moves on to all the other varied experiences that compose her life, she will be able to bring with her a feeling of satisfaction and completion about what has been, whether it involved great joy or great sorrow. She was fully there in that moment, whether she experienced it as being painful, joyous, sad or miraculous.

This very moment, when experienced fully with all our sensation, feeling and thought, becomes eternal. We will remember it fully because we are truly here. If we are entangled with churning automatic thoughts in the background of our minds, we will not fully perceive the present moment. If small waves of worry about past and future events are washing over us while we read, the new material coming in will not be fully digested. So, in the next moment, we have undigested material to deal with as well as the new present moment, and we remain stuck in a labyrinth of undigested experience. The only possibility we have is to separate ourselves from these churning thoughts, these background feelings, and make an effort to be fully present, now. We can do nothing about the past. It is what it is. We know nothing about the future because it is dependent on the now, on this very moment. The only thing that is real is now.

We may also allow our experience to be stolen from us as a result of our own lack of preparation and naivety. We are responsible for our attitude to the events that life brings us. If we meet an experience with a resigned attitude, we will become victims. If we are aware that the way women are encouraged to give birth in hospital is not quite right, but fail to act upon this awareness, then we share some responsibility for the outcome of our birth. To act upon it might be to research home birth or to search for a teaching that offers guidance.

If we do not yet realize that our attitude determines our experiences, then it does not matter, but the moment we become aware of it, time begins to count. From that point on, we become responsible for our attitude. We can no longer be merely victims of circumstance, because we know and understand what can be done. Birth and death mark the major transitions in our lives. Of course, it is important to strive to be present in all of life's moments, but the momentous event of giving birth is on such a scale that we actually take it seriously and attempt to prepare. All women know instinctively that this is one of the ultimate objectives of their bodies: a unique opportunity to be fully present in the complete unfolding of idea into matter, of infusing matter with life force.

Conscious labour

Birth is a noun. Labour is also a verb, something that is ongoing and that requires effort, a process, not an isolated event or a concept. In the beginning was the verb. Everything is process. Even rocks are born, live and die. A step on the way towards conscious labour is to try to see the whole, the entire process that is birthing. This includes pregnancy and breastfeeding. To view the birth as an isolated incident robs it of its full potential. Birth can be said to begin about forty days before the due date, when my 'usual self' gradually begins to turn inwards to allow instinctive function to come to the fore. Birth ends about forty days after a woman's due date, when her womb has returned to its normal size and she has recovered from the physical effects of birth and established an emotional bond with her baby.

To understand this better, it helps to understand the concept of hyperintention. Hyperintention is when only the peak of a process unfolding is experienced, leaving out the build-up and the wind-down. A clear example which most women will be familiar with is when lovemaking becomes only an orgasm with no foreplay preceding it and no post-coital tenderness to follow it.

To let go of hyperintention is to experience life more fully. If you go away on holiday, it is not only the week that you are away which comprises the experience. The full experience includes choosing where to go, planning the route, buying the tickets and the state of anticipation and excitement that goes with it. It also includes the return home, with new impressions that make you see familiar things in a different light and the experiences of your holiday that enrich your everyday life.

The way most women in the west give birth today, taken out of our ordinary environment and familiar surroundings and placed almost in an operating theatre, is hyperintended in the extreme. We can strive to round off the edges of our birth — to not allow it to become pointy and sharp. The waves of life's experiences are rolling, not jagged. They have a beginning, a middle and an end. If we stop chasing the peak experience we may be able to start living.

It is the same with birth. Birth is not a single event, an isolated peak. It is a *triad*, a whole, comprised of three initiations: pregnancy, childbirth and breastfeeding. This is the holy trinity of bringing life into the world.

In my native tongue, Swedish, a pregnant woman is said to be in 'the blessed state' — *Det välsignade tillståndet*. She is in a state of grace, allowed for a short time to make contact, through her body, with the real world that lies beyond time and matter. The life force moves through her body, through the tissues she has prepared for it, and is able to enter the three-dimensional world that we know through her. It shows. She glows, she smiles like Mona Lisa, her hair shines, her eyes sparkle. She is blessed amongst women.

2. Conception

Making space for a child

In order for something to be received you first need a receptacle. The essence of a jug is not its outer china structure, but the empty space it contains. This is not just about ensuring that there is physical space for a child, although this is part of it too. Is there room in your life for a child? If you make sure there is, it will help your child to be able to come, for you to become pregnant. To do this, you need to think about making the necessary space and time in your life that a child would occupy.

Look at your home and ask yourself: what would be needed for a child to live in this environment? It is not necessary to refurbish your home or to decorate one room to use as a nursery. Is the way you live child-friendly? Would you be stressed by an infant vomiting on your expensive carpet? Is your home full of precious ornaments? Would you find it awkward walking around your house with your crying newborn in the dark, rocking her to sleep on your shoulder? Because this is sure to happen.

Look at how you live and ask yourself: am I short of time? Look at what you do with your time, what your day is filled with. If you want a child to be in your life you will need to clear out some of the old things. You can do it now, intentionally, in advance, to make space for your baby, or you can be pushed into doing this because of the constant demands of a baby.

Look at the direction of your life and ask yourself: where am I heading? Your child will be the main influence on how your outer life, and potentially also your inner, transformative work, is structured for a long time to come, perhaps twenty years. It is possible to use your creative powers to prepare for aligning the direction of your life, inner and outer, with the upbringing of your child. Perhaps either you or your partner can work from home. Maybe you can move to an environment more suitable for children, which also proves cheaper, so one of you can stay at home. Refrain from seeing caring for your child as another chore, a job to be done. Looking after your child is a great honour and a privilege and should be assigned its due place in your life.

As a Buddhist monk once advised a young couple trying to conceive a child, it is necessary to do two things: fuck and pray. Neither one alone can make a person come into the world, even if we are encouraged to think so by the pervading dogma of contemporary science. Perhaps you have never prayed, yet have conceived a child. Well, not all prayers are heard by ourselves. It is in our subconscious mind that all our essential wishes are spoken.

Discuss your options with your doctor, or healing practitioner, and do your own research. Take responsibility for your situation. Living from the position of being a victim of circumstance only conjures up suffering.

If the child you long for does not come, it may be that your highest aim in life is to transform precisely that experience. It is possible to create your reality rather than to allow yourself to be a passive victim of circumstance. Don't let yourself be trapped in the fast-flowing current of life like a dead fish. The living swim upstream and are, through their efforts, able to fulfil their highest purpose.

I wish to be me

You are the chosen one.

You are the one in 360,000,000 who made it, who didn't give up, didn't falter and was committed to the end. You are the living result of the selection of the very best, most able and determined. What happened to that dynamic? It rightfully belongs to you.

Dormant you lie, in your mother's ovary, waiting, waiting for the moment, your moment, to come. You are released and travel down the fallopian tube, hoping, waiting silently, patiently, passively for your lover, who is active, struggling, battling, swimming, working, expending himself in his quest for you — quiet round perfection, white as the moon, you lie, waiting.

In the moment you meet, the neutralizing force of life enters and joins the active and the passive, transforming you both. Lost forever is your passive and his active nature, you are now one, the new, a growing, living whole. You have joined and become potential man.

In the waves and spasms of orgasm you enter the human race. Out of the ecstasy of creation you come.

You only had a 50/50 chance of being born as only half of all fertilized eggs survive all the way through pregnancy: you made it. What was it that you wanted so much to come here for?

You came here because you wished to. You had the choice and you made it, whole-heartedly, willingly. You will come again. You knew what awaited you. You knew the difficulties you would face in this life. You knew, and intentionally, having decided in advance, you came. You begged to be born.

Your parents', daily lives were on a different level from yours, the level of ordinary consciousness, of waking sleep. In the ecstasy of orgasm, love and pleasure intermingled and gave them a foretaste of what is rightfully theirs. The real world. That is where they were able to connect with the place where you resided. You were offered an opening; you were invited in. You knew what you would lose and what you had to gain. You came.

Your mortal coil unfolds in your mother's womb. Your presence is still voluntary and intentional. You are needed as the life force that oversees the unfurling. You provide the spirit of life.

Your effort, care, attention and love infuse and nurture this automatically-doubling matter into a spiritualized being.

You grow yourself a body. You, the life force, enter matter and animate it, you structure and pace and control its growth and development.

This is the fire of life, electricity with all three parts present, not only the positive and negative poles such as we have become accustomed to know it. This electricity of life begins to flicker between neurones. You compose your body. You attract, arrange, organize matter.

You reside deep within the centre and act as the anchor, the centre of gravity around which matter can accumulate. You coat yourself in automatically-growing matter. You attract your body through your will to come into being. You are the invisible, the unmanifest core. The still centre of the whirling dervish. The eye of the storm. The I of the storm. The word becoming manifest.

You come and go as you please. You may choose to abandon the project at any time. You chose to stay.

> *At the still point of the turning world. Neither flesh nor fleshless;*
> *Neither from nor towards; at the still point, there the dance is,*
> *But neither arrest nor movement. And do not call it fixity,*
> *Where past and future are gathered. Neither movement from*
>   *nor towards,*
> *Neither ascent nor decline. Except for the point, the still point,*
> *There would be no dance, and there is only the dance.*
> (From 'Burnt Norton,' *Four Quartets*, T.S. Eliot)

Conception

As the 360 million or so sperm race towards the egg after ejaculation, they are not all blindly trying to get there first. Some sperm take on the function of blocking the cervical canal so that the sperm of another man cannot enter. Others take on the role of smoothing the passage through the tissues of the womb and fallopian tubes, filling the nooks and crevices and lining the path like sentries. Each one plays its role fully to allow a sperm the best possible chance of reaching the egg.

The sperm is the smallest cell in the human body, the egg the largest. An egg is about 100,000 times heavier than the sperm. A woman's eggs were all made while she was still in her mother's womb. Half of what provides a baby's body has been ready and waiting since the birth of its own mother. A newborn girl already has all the 360 or so fully-formed eggs she will release later in life, some of which may be fertilized and become her children. A male foetus is already producing the sperm that will eventually fertilize the egg.

While maturing in the fallopian tube, your egg will exile half of its 46 chromosomes to a polar body, leaving 23 chromosomes in the centre of the egg that is eventually released during ovulation. The same halving occurs in each sperm, but here the result is two separate sperm with 23 chromosomes each. 23 chromosomes from the mother and 23 chromosomes from the father make the 46 chromosomes of the new individual. A single chromosome in the sperm will determine the gender of your child.

Each chromosome contains two metres of DNA. Only 1.5 % of the genes contained in these two metres of instructions make us human. We share half of our genes with fruit flies and one third with daffodils.

So what, then, is it that makes us so different?

Our potential.

Man is seed incarnate. We have higher functions that we can only access by working on and perfecting ourselves. The many ways of spiritual development that have appeared over the millennia around the world have such self-perfecting as their aim, for example the teachings of the Sufis, the Essenes, Tibetan Buddhists, Alchemists, Cabbalists and the ancient Egyptian religion. It is by transforming our psychology, our inner world, from a base level of appetites and pleasure-seeking, that we can become truly normal, to become created in the image of God, or as Adam before the Fall. This is what is meant by the biblical saying that the kingdom of heaven lies within. We have the potential to become normal, which is not the same as the usual or commonplace. We have the opportunity to truly fulfil our potential.

It takes several hours for the sperm to swim the 15–18 cm to the fallopian tube. Many get lost in the dead ends, cavities and mazes that comprise the lining of the uterus, the womb and fallopian tubes. During their journey up the vagina and through the uterus, the sperm are influenced by the new environment and are gradually transformed by substances in the tissues they pass over: the sperm become 'capacitated' and are now able to penetrate and fertilize the egg.

During ovulation the mucus of the uterus and womb is especially runny, which makes it easier for the sperm to swim its way through the woman's passages and reach the egg. It has to get through the mucal plug that protects the uterus from infection. The woman's own white blood cells will attack and kill any sperm they come into contact with. The rate of attrition is extremely high: an ejaculation containing a million sperm would not be enough to have a chance of fertilizing the egg. If the sperm run out of energy on their way to the egg, they are able to refuel from the secretions in the fallopian tube. A thousand beats with its tail propel the sperm about one centimetre. The sperm have to swim against the current of cilia, which are tiny, hair-like protrusions that line the fallopian tube. About one hundred of the original 360 million will make it as far as the egg.

Once the winning sperm has entered the egg, it loses its tail and a chemical process seals the outer coating of the egg to all other sperm. However, those sperm that have already reached the egg and burrowed part of their way in to it will remain. These sperm do not lose their tails and they keep on burrowing, their tails beating and turning in a spiral. This halo of wiggling sperm tails allows the egg to begin to rotate anticlockwise and facilitates its progress down the fallopian tube.

The material body is grown out of matter from your genetic parents. Two becomes three: two cells make a third, a new whole.

The evolution of the foetus follows the same mathematical laws of unfurling, spiralling and growth that govern all processes in the universe: in the beginning was the Word, the idea, spirit without form. The foetus differentiates and comes into being in the three-dimensional world of space and time. From the one, the new whole of the fertilized egg, spring two, the dyad. Out of two come many. Four. Eight. Sixteen. Thirty-two. Holy doubling.

In the beginning was the Word, and the Word was with God,
and the Word was God. (John 1:1)

I am One that transforms
   into Two,
I am Two that transforms
   into Four,
I am Four that transforms
   into Eight.
After this I am One again.
(Egyptian, Hermopolitan, creation myth)

3. Pregnancy

Growth of the foetus

The first cell division takes place one day after fertilization. After four to five days the new life is divided in two again, into embryo and placenta. At this stage, all cells are identical. Every one of them holds the potential to become one of two hundred types of cells and is known by contemporary science as stem cells.

Like these cells, we all have the potential to become what we were really meant to be, to fulfil the higher purpose intended for us. Your highest potential is not the same as my highest potential. Each one of us has a unique and vital function to perform. We don't know it yet. When you start to wake up to this reality you have the possibility of preparing to become what you have come here for: to become your Self.

The cells lie in waiting, dividing samely, waiting for the Word that starts the process of specialization in them. They may become liver cells, expert at filtering toxins from the blood. They may become brain cells, sparks of understanding and responsibility in the mind. They may become heart cells, contracting and pumping ceaselessly for your allocated 72 years of potential transformation. They may become bone cells, upholding your structure rigidly so that you may walk, and live, and act. They may become skin cells, forming the barrier between inside and outside the fortress, jealously guarded by the white blood cells whose first question is always: friend or foe? They may become red blood cells who are over here, over there, never anywhere in particular, ceaselessly spreading the daily bread around the temple.

Every single cell of this first life has the potential to perform any one of these highly specialized and complex cell functions. Why does such a cell become a liver cell? How can we come to know what our highest destiny is, so that we may fulfil it?

After seven days of travelling, the ball of cells reaches the uterus, its room, its universe for the next nine months. It anchors itself to the wall of the womb by sugar molecules that protrude from its surface and hook on to similar molecules in the lining of the womb. The ovary then starts producing progesterone, which sends a signal to the pituitary gland that pregnancy is underway and that the foreign body, the baby, must not be expelled. The new life also produces chemicals that weaken the mother's immune system locally, in the womb.

Taking great care over several days, the growing clump selects a place to embed itself in the womb. It will try to find a spot near the top of the womb, but sometimes it has to make do with a lower position, which can give rise to complications during birth, when the placenta blocks the child's exit. Once the new life has attached itself to the lining of the womb it begins to interact with the mother's tissues. Hormones produced by the new life enter the mother's bloodstream, allowing us to read the results of a pregnancy test.

The new life also emits signals that ensure that the mucus in the womb becomes thicker, making it easier for the embryo to stay firmly attached. A thick mucal plug blocks the entrance to the womb to ensure its integrity. The embryo also influences the muscles of the womb hormonally, making them softer and more elastic. This is a critical period in the development of the new life. If any part of the process is left incomplete or occurs in the wrong sequence the entire lining of the womb will be expelled, as during a normal period.

In the first octave, up to the point where the clump reaches eight cells, all cells are identical in appearance and function. By the time the clump is eight days old and has reached a mass of about a hundred cells, the cells begin to differentiate. The individual cells start to look different and begin to perform different functions. Every twelve hours the cells divide.

During the second week, the nerve cells begin to take form. Electricity surges through the clump of matter, the life force flickers through the neurones. These differentiating cells gradually start to reach out towards each other and eventually a connection is made. The new nerve cells then begin to communicate and the first systems are tested. Each minute 2,500,000 nerve cells are made. Nerve cells are made during gestation and remain the same throughout life.

During the third week the ball of cells folds in on itself to form a long tube. The top of this tube will become the head, the lower part will become the trunk of the body. The arms and legs then bud from this trunk.

The cells that have been allocated the function of heart will have reached critical mass. They sense each other's presence and readiness, and at the given moment, one of them spontaneously contracts, triggering those nearby, which trigger cells adjacent to them, and so on, until all heart cells are beating together, beating as one. They work in unison, towards the same aim, ceaselessly, in order to realize their highest potential.

The eye develops from a stalk protruding from the brain tissue. The ear is formed from three parts: brain tissue becomes the inner ear with its organ of equilibrium and hearing. The outer ear comes a little later and the middle ear develops from a protrusion in the throat to form the ossicles: the hammer, anvil and stirrup.

In week four, the embryo differentiates into three layers of tissue: an outer layer, 'ectoderm,' which is destined to become your baby's brain and nervous system, as well as the skin, hair, teeth and nails; a middle layer, 'mesoderm,' destined to become your baby's muscles, skeleton, heart and blood vessels, the lymph nodes as well as the ovaries, testicles and kidneys; an inner layer, 'endoderm,' destined to become your baby's bowels, urinary tract and lungs.

After eight weeks, the embryo becomes known as a foetus, meaning 'young one' in Latin. This is because all organs are now formed, although still developing. The first octave is completed and she may enter our cosmos, our scale, and is now a living body like ours, only smaller. She has made the transition from the microcosmos, the world of cells, to our cosmos, the world of the body.

The first seven months of pregnancy develop and test all systems, and the last six weeks of pregnancy provide time for building up a layer of fat under the skin, in preparation for life outside the womb. The foetus steadily gains weight at a rate of about two hundred grams per week.

The placenta

At eight weeks the placenta is mature and replaces the yolk sack on which the embryo relied for the first two months. The placenta is unique to mammals and acts as an exchange between the foetus' and the mother's blood.

The placenta serves as a filter through which nutrients enter the foetus' bloodstream and waste products are returned to the mother's blood, where they are processed by her fully-formed vital organs. The placenta also releases the hormones that cause morning sickness. These hormones prevent the mother's immune system from rejecting the foreign body that it is nurturing.

The mother's blood vessels enter into the placenta and disappear into its depths in narrower and narrower channels. The baby's umbilical cord disappears into the placenta, becoming narrower and narrower. Microscopic protrusions from the umbilical vein and arteries known as a chorionic villi act as super-fine blood vessels through which the foetus' blood flows. Only a thin membrane separates the two blood systems. Oxygen, nutrients and other substances can pass from the mother's blood and enter the foetus' bloodstream through this membrane. The foetus' blood cells release waste products which pass through the membrane into the mother's blood to be disposed of.

A few foetal cells are present in a pregnant woman's blood, and the baby's DNA circulates in the mother's bloodstream. Presence within presence. The two of you, mother and child, are as one. Blood relations.

In the placenta, two totally separate blood supplies connect and an exchange of substances between two living beings takes place. A continuous direct exchange proceeds throughout the pregnancy. This is the beginning of the development of emotional function and occurs only in mammals. Animals that lay eggs — birds and reptiles — are biologically separate from their young, sometimes even before the egg is fertilized. They develop no emotional function and have only instinctive function. Emotional function is the preserve of mammals.

Anyone who has cared for horses or dogs will recognize that we share this with them. They can show us what a pure emotional function can be like. Dogs and horses do not exhibit negative emotion (instinctive reactions such as aggression or fear, fight or flight, are not truly emotions, nor is mourning a negative emotion: it is a healthy response to loss). Animals do not become indignant and are incapable of regret. This is our birthright too, but the child imitates the negative emotions of those around him from an early age and soon becomes proficient.

The special emotional connection you have with your mother is a result of the direct part she played in developing your emotional function, and this begins in the placenta.

Building emotional function

Mammals are those animals that gestate their young inside the body and that suckle their young. This develops a particular, biological closeness and contact between mother and young which is the seed of their emotional life. In this way, there is no difference between a human and a cow, say. Both have an emotional function developed by gestation and suckling. However, humans are different from any other animal in having an intellectual function. It is worth emphasizing that this is one of our most dormant functions, and is not to be confused with practical problem solving or the right/wrong progressive dichotomies we generally call thinking.

When in the womb, the foetus shares all the mother's emotions and bio-chemical reactions. When you are stressed you produce the stress hormone cortisol. When you are happy you produce endorphins, natural pleasure chemicals. When you are relaxed you produce a substance that resembles tranquillizers. All these chemicals permeate your entire system and communicate with every part of your body, through the circulatory system of the blood.

Physiologically, the mother's heart rate and blood pressure are directly affected by her emotional state. Every cell in your body is affected by such neurophysiological changes. Your moods, reactions and feelings are translated into the chemical language that flows through your bloodstream. The word is made flesh. An idea which has no three-dimensional body is given form through the chemical responses of your body and becomes manifest in the three-dimensional world. Here, it can be transformed into action, through the organized, spiritualized matter we call the body.

Messenger molecules such as adrenaline, noradrenaline, oxytocin and serotonin pass through the placenta and elicit a response in the baby. The influence these chemical messengers have on you, your feelings, are also felt by the unborn child.

Children born to mothers who endure extreme stress during pregnancy can experience mental problems in later life. Stress and anxiety in pregnancy increase the mother's own levels of cortisol, and this is then passed on to the unborn baby, affecting its own stress response system. Anxiety in pregnancy is associated with higher levels of the stress hormone cortisol in children. High levels of cortisol are associated with psychological problems such as depression and anxiety. Extreme stress during pregnancy could affect the child's stress response system, known as the hypothalamic pituitary adrenal axis.

When you carry a baby in your womb, it is enveloped in your cosmos. Your feelings are law for the foetus. There is no other world beyond that of Mother. The baby lies enveloped and saturated in your emotions. The baby's emotional function is born out of your emotional function. Lying in the womb is an extended practice period for developing such an independent function outside the womb.

This is an opportunity for you, the mother, to be more vigilant and send negative thoughts back to the ether from which they come. We are free to do so at any time, but pregnancy might help us to be a little more alert for the sake of our unborn child.

Dispelling negative thoughts

We are brought up to believe that negative feelings are generated from within ourselves. We are hypnotized by all the influences around us, such as the pervasive negative reporting of the media and the negative emotional states we have been shown by role models during our upbringing. We are conditioned to think that it is our duty to feel bad about certain things, to watch the news and to keep up with suffering that we can do nothing about.

However, it is possible to let a negative feeling pass you by, rather than catch it on one of the many 'hooks' our upbringing has constructed in our psyche. Begin to draw these artificially constructed hooks in when a negative thought comes and you will not catch it.

If we look at nature, we can see that everything has a purpose, from the jagged edges of a leaf to the huge ears of an elephant. Evolution and the intelligence of creation are extremely efficient and nothing is wasted. It is the same in man. The secretion of the bonding hormone oxytocin when we touch another human being bonds us together. The release of adrenaline when confronted with danger prepares us to run fast or to fight for our lives. These are examples of our instinctive function creating emotional responses that we experience as feelings. Negative emotions such as irritation, worry or feelings of injustice serve no purpose in nature. These negative emotions consume energy that we need for the effective functioning of our organism. If we observe our expression of negative emotions over time, we will see that they do not come from ourselves but are triggered by external events. The expression of negative emotions is so commonplace as to be considered 'normal' by most. If we look at the world's spiritual teachings we see that one of the steps on the way to self-improvement is to become aware of habitual subconscious negative emotions, a step towards becoming free of the power we allow them to hold over us.

We are not obliged to take irritation, indignation, self-pity, worry, resentment or regret on board and allow it to permeate our system. Let it go. Throw it to the wind. You were never intended to carry that burden around.

Twins

There is extensive evidence of the exceptionally strong connection between twins that endures through life, and many examples of twins who have married at the same time, had children around the same time and even died at the same time.

Twins share the same conditions while in the womb: they both exchange substances with their mother's blood during the same period of her life, both live enveloped in her cloud of emotion. Both are then (in normal conditions) breastfed during the affirmation period of the fledgling emotional function, by the same mother, in similar circumstances and experiencing similar emotional conditions. Twins share the same emotional function, and they remain connected throughout life, whether the adult person is aware of it or not. They have been built in the same way, under the same conditions, biologically and emotionally.

Identical twins also share the same genetic make-up. Non-identical twins share emotional function but their genetic make-up differs. The ancient science of human typology can provide many answers that contemporary science has not yet formulated.

Hormonal changes and increased receptivity

The mood fluctuations resulting from hormonal changes are a form of heightened awareness. All women will have had a taste of this in the days around their period. We become more open, sensitive, cry more easily and recognize the things that are wrong about the way we live, our mechanicalism, more easily. We do not become more irritable, which is how an abnormal world perceives our behaviour; we become more sensitive.

Most psychological disciplines recognize the reality of the inner child, that part of our selves which remains unchanged since childhood. In some disciplines it is also known as the essence of a person, that which is truly ours. The outer layer is then known as personality, that which is learned. In most cases essence stops growing in childhood as it is not stimulated or even recognized by those around us. Personality is encouraged and its growth is aided further by schooling and education.

Take the opportunity that pregnancy provides to strive to heal unresolved emotional issues and improve your communication with those that are close to you. You will find yourself more open and more ready to acknowledge the difficulties that lie between you and your loved ones. You are more sensitive, more receptive, you can see the world of emotion more clearly and can recognize what is wrong in it.

After you have given birth, this gift will gradually subside and you will return to your usual state, in which you don't 'make such a big deal of things,' you are not so 'over-sensitive' and when you are more happy with the usual way of interacting and living again. But this sensitivity is a blessing. You see the world more clearly now, you have the opportunity to try to mend what is broken. And you can't begin to do this until you are able to acknowledge that something is wrong.

Acknowledge and accept your feelings. If things are not as they should be, see it, know it. It doesn't necessarily mean that you will be able to change it, at least not straight away. If we pretend that everything is fine as it is, then we remove the potential for development. This period of openness may be a first step towards becoming your Self.

You are likely to find that the relationship with your own mother changes or intensifies when you become pregnant. You can finally understand her in a biological way, understand what she did for you and the hardships she experienced so that you might live. You may also begin to recognize what her shortcomings were while carrying you and when you were very young.

Your relationship with your mother comes to the fore and other relationships take on less significance during this period. Although this may be painful, it is a priceless opportunity for mother and daughter to reconnect, accept and understand each other more deeply. Later, after the birth, your life will start spinning at the speed required for dealing with nappies, feeding, soothing, washing, cooking and so on and this opportunity will be gone. Make the most of it now, in your wondrous open state of emotional receptivity. Blessed art thou amongst women.

You are now experiencing being a living link in the great chain of heredity: you are passing on genetic material, habits and dynamics and you have an opportunity to influence what is passed on.

This depends on your knowledge of yourself. Do you know what you might pass on? Can you see yourself, objectively, from outside, as you seem to others? Not as it appears from within, looking out at the world through your eyes. By becoming aware of yourself and how generations-old habits manifest through you, you can know what you might pass on. By knowing yourself you have an opportunity to repair the past and prepare the future.

Hysteria

Hysteria comes from the Latin word for womb. This can be seen clearly in the word hysterectomy, for example, which is the medical term for the removal of the womb. What is hysteria? In our language it has become associated with the outbursts of over-emotional women. But if we look a little deeper into the meaning that lies behind the word, what is it really? It is the ability to make something out of nothing. It is encapsulated in English in the expression 'to make a mountain out of a molehill.'

For every phenomenon, it might be said that there is a threefold possibility of manifestation: manifesting in its degenerated form, manifesting in its neutral form and manifesting in its refined form. Hysteria, then, in its degenerated form, is indeed the over-emotional and uncontrolled outbursts of women, making far too much out of nothing. In its neutral form, hysteria is the organ of generation, the womb, fulfilling its biological function of making something out of nothing. In its highest, refined form, hysteria is the woman's directed creative ability, intuition. This is quite different from the creative ability of imagination. Intuition involves 'seeing' with all three parts of you at once, with the physical body, with emotion and with the intellect. Then our net for catching cues from the world around us can be cast much wider and we can see that which is not yet known. We can make something out of nothing.

However, due to our abnormal enjoyment of negative emotions, negative associations have become attached to the expression 'hysteria.' Think about it for a minute. To make a mountain out of a molehill is no mean feat. And it is a creative ability unique to woman. In the context of birth, it is the ability to create and maintain life.

You have this wonderful organ within you that can create the conditions required for life to arise. It can then nurture and encourage this spark of life so that a healthy, complete, complex organism may emerge into the world. Your womb, hysteria, is empty, clean, lying silent, ready and waiting, never forgetting what it is meant to do when the time comes.

It lies ready to apply exactly the right amount of increasing pressure on the foetus during childbirth. It lies ready to reciprocally communicate with your pituitary gland so that tiny droplets of oxytocin are transmitted at the ideal intervals for mother and child, maximising rest and recovery while ensuring expedient progress down the birth canal. It lies ready to let go of the placenta at just the right moment and contract back to its pear-shaped size again, in preparation for next time.

It lies silent within you, knowing all it is capable of, yet waiting always for your word. It doesn't rush, it doesn't stop prematurely, it doesn't compromise its integrity, it doesn't exert too much pressure, or too little. Next time someone calls you hysterical, you can respond with a Mona Lisa smile that knows.

Instinctive function and morning sickness

During pregnancy, the mother's blood volume leaps by up to fifty per cent in order to supply the baby with sufficient oxygen. Her heart works and pumps and beats, ceaselessly, tirelessly, and assumes full responsibility for the critical function it performs, nurturing not only the being of its primary service, but also creating the conditions for another being to enter the world.

The mother's lungs increase their capacity to absorb up to twenty per cent more oxygen than normal in the last three months of pregnancy. You have a unique opportunity to observe the workings of your instinctive part and how its intelligence operates during pregnancy.

The instinctive function also manifests itself in cravings and aversions. Some foods become irresistible and it is possible to observe how your child builds itself a body from say oranges or potatoes. These foods contain exactly the nutrients, minerals and vitamins needed at that particular stage and this is communicated to your instinctive function. If you have not become completely out of tune with your instinctive needs by overriding them repeatedly, such as we do when smoking or drinking alcohol to excess, you will know exactly what you need to eat.

Nausea or morning sickness is the result of your heightened sensitivity and being more in tune with your instinctive function. This ensures that there is no chance of you eating bad food that might harm the foetus, which is at a particularly sensitive stage of development during the early part of pregnancy.

Some women suffer from severe nausea during pregnancy and it can get progressively worse each time. You may try everything — ginger, orange juice, sucking a lemon, getting your partner to bring you a cracker and a cup of sweet tea first thing in the morning, eating frequent small snacks, using anti-travel sickness bracelets with pressure points on your wrist, acupuncture — and still find that nothing works. It may be that the sickness does not subside until after you have given birth, when it just vanishes, which can be quite surprising. You may have been feeling sick for so long that you had almost grown used to it.

Acceptance might be a more constructive approach, but that's easy to say when you are no longer experiencing overwhelming nausea 24 hours a day. The case described above is extreme, but they do occur. Many women feel nauseous for the first three months, and improve in the latter stages of pregnancy. There are also women who experience no nausea at all, so if that's you, count yourself lucky!

Although this condition has been carefully studied, contemporary science is still not certain what causes it. However, it has been observed that women who suffer from morning sickness have a substantially lower risk of miscarriage and stillbirth than those who do not. Some reports also suggest that nausea is associated with fewer premature deliveries, higher birth weights, reduced birth defects and improved survival of infants. Instinctive function is put on a higher level of alert so as to avoid food poisoning or the accidental ingestion of toxins, which might not harm the mother but could prove critical to the unborn child's development.

It has also been found that mothers who feel sick during the first few months of pregnancy, eat less and therefore gain less weight in the early stages of pregnancy. Less weight gain in the first trimester allows the placenta to grow more, and the placenta, of course, supplies blood to the developing foetus. When the mother starts eating more again as the nausea subsides, the baby also puts on weight and can be adequately supplied by a healthy, large placenta.

You may not be able to abide coffee, alcohol, cigarettes and many other things which you usually consume, having overridden instinctive function for long enough for it to have become subdued. A revulsion towards some strong tastes and scents, such as garlic, may be your instinctive function showing you that they contain potent chemicals. Listen to what it wants to tell you.

Your moving function

Moving function relates to those automatic movements that do not require the continuous participation of the intellect, but which have to be learned. This includes all routine movements, such as handwriting, once your intellect no longer needs to be engaged in shaping the letters or connecting them together. When you first learned to write, your intellectual centre was involved, and you gradually trained your moving centre to take over the task. It now proceeds automatically.

Intellectual centre is much slower than moving centre. Try to remember your experience of learning to cycle. At first your intellectual centre controls your movements, and the process is slow and laborious. Eventually your moving centre learns what to do and begins to take over. You no longer involve your intellectual centre in every push of the pedal, steering or balancing.

The intelligence of your moving centre operates independently. We can even read using only our moving centre. Most of us can recall times when we have suddenly 'woken up' (engaged our intellectual centre) to find that we have read two or three pages without having any idea of the content. Our moving centre has scanned the letters, taken in the words and even connected sentences, but this centre is not capable of taking in meaning. For this to happen, the intellectual centre needs to be involved. There are many more examples. Try to find some for yourself, from your own experience.

For the purposes of pregnancy, it may be helpful to become more aware of your moving centre — to observe what it does that is helpful or not helpful to your current state. Observe yourself and start to recognize patterns of movement that belong to your moving centre. Perhaps you automatically bend down to pick things up from the floor without flexing your knees and keeping your back straight. Now is an excellent time to become aware of this.

During pregnancy your bones become more flexible and pliable to allow your child to pass easily through the birth canal. After the birth of your child, you will be carrying this increasingly heavy bundle for many hours a day and will frequently be picking your baby up, sometimes urgently, to avoid danger. Prepare for the future by becoming aware of your moving patterns now. Many women experience back problems during pregnancy and after giving birth. Becoming more aware of your automatic movements will help you to avoid unnecessary difficulties later.

Sex

Sexual arousal during pregnancy can be wonderfully easy to come by. The hormonal changes coupled with the pressure on your vulva and pubic mound from the weight of the growing womb means that you may find yourself ready and up for it most of the time. Enjoy! Sex during pregnancy will not harm the baby. However, it is important to know that during the last two weeks of pregnancy sex can trigger labour. You can use this as your own natural induction if your baby exceeds its due date and you want to help the process along.

Miscarriage

Miscarriage can be caused by a number of different factors: if something goes wrong in the unfolding process of the new life, in the division of cells, or if there is damage to a chromosome; if several sperm reach the egg at once and more chromosome matter than required enters the egg; or if the chromosomes in the sperm that entered the egg are damaged or poor. Sperm is more often the cause of an early miscarriage than the egg. The egg might also get caught in the tissues of the fallopian tube and be prevented from entering the womb, and if the egg becomes attached there, the result is an ectopic pregnancy, which cannot be completed.

The children lost are perhaps those who were unprepared, who were not quite ready to come. Perhaps the matter assigned to them had some imperfection and a decision was made to abort the attempt — a withered limb, an imperfect heart. Who knows? These lost children are lost only in our limited three-dimensional understanding. The being you call your baby chooses to come and chooses to go. Strive to respect that choice and wait for the conditions to be right.

A period of physical readjustment to prepare your womb for conception again is absolutely necessary, and so is a period of psychological recovery or mourning. In order to recover you will need to give these processes the time they take, otherwise you will carry the pain deep inside you until you choose to address it, and this may make you ill in other ways.

Each miscarriage will need a period of about six months for the body and mind to readjust. You may need longer, but hardly a shorter period. During this period you need not necessarily change your outward behaviour that much, although your body may require rest and gentle treatment for a while.

However, the time needs to be allocated and you may feel sad, tired, an aching, and a longing. Strive to accept this; it is part of healing. Eventually the wound may start to itch, you will find the sensation of hurt less deep and the wound will close. You will always carry a scar, as you will after each and every unique birth. Carry your scars with pride, think of them as your battle scars, the marks that remind you of how you became a woman, a mother and more wise.

Down's syndrome and amniocentesis

Down's syndrome is caused by an extra chromosome that interferes with the development of the other chromosomes. In children with Down's syndrome, emotional function appears fully developed and can be extra sensitive. Although there are difficulties resulting from having a child with this condition, it can also be a gift if you can see it and nurture it in the right way. For example, perhaps your child will have the ability to express a state, an emotional understanding, through music that a 'normal' person can't.

Amniocentesis involves inserting a needle into the foetal sack, puncturing it, and extracting some amniotic fluid in order to obtain the foetus' DNA. There is a risk associated with this and in some cases the procedure generates a miscarriage. Before you embark on any test to see if your baby has Down's syndrome or a major disability you need to address the possibility that the test is positive. What then? What will you do? How might you feel? Tread carefully when you try to know the future: what seems like a blessing may be a curse and what seems like a curse may be a blessing in disguise.

When something goes 'wrong,' it is not the outer event that ought to be changed, but our inner state which responds to it. If we can build inner balance, we will no longer be blown over by the slightest gust, whether 'good' or 'bad.' We will always have some part of ourselves that is not at the mercy of outside chance events.

There is a well-known Chinese tale that goes as follows. A man owns a horse. One night the horse runs away. The next morning his neighbours commiserate with him: 'What a shame that you should lose your handsome stallion.' 'We shall see,' replies the man. The next night, the horse returns, bringing with it a young filly. The next morning, his neighbours congratulate him: 'What good luck. Not only has your stallion returned, but now you have two good horses.' 'We shall see,' says the man. The next day his son goes horse riding and, in an unfortunate fall, breaks his arm. The next day, the man's neighbours commiserate with him: 'What an unfortunate accident, that your son should break his arm in this way.' 'We shall see,' says the man. The next day, a royal envoy arrives to round up all the young men in the neighbourhood to go to war, sparing only the sick and injured. Again, the man's neighbours congratulate him: 'What good luck, that your son should avoid having to go to war in this way.' 'We shall see ...' says the man.

IVF and fertility treatment

Do everything you can to conceive naturally and do it wholeheartedly. If you still don't conceive then completely let go of Plan A and feel no regret. Then attempt wholeheartedly to conceive with IVF, but set yourself a time limit so that you do not become consumed by the attempt and let IVF hijack your life. Give it, say, one year or three courses of treatment. Or proceed with the process of adopting a child, equally whole-heartedly.

If you are not able to have a child by any means, then let it go completely. As hard as it may be, you will then need to focus on transforming your experience of not having a child. 'Take hold tightly, let go lightly.' (A.R. Orage, *On Love*)

4. Preparing for Childbirth

Preparing your tissues

Your tissues will work for your and your child's benefit in an unprecedented manner during labour. They have never done it before, yet they know exactly what to do and have waited silently for this moment all your life. Your job is largely to get out of the way of the natural functioning of your tissues and organs during childbirth.

This is counter to the way we are usually brought up to live our lives. We are constantly urged to do more, be more active, to take control, to fill our time. Mastery, adulthood, responsibility as a human being, as a woman, includes knowing what your instinctive parts do infinitely better than 'you' do.

In order to be able to respond, rather than react, to your tissues and smooth the way for their work, you need to establish a connection with them. With patient effort you will be amazed at the range of sensation available to you.

Make space for your preparation for birth. You will need a physical space where you can be sure you will be undisturbed for thirty minutes or so, preferably the space where you intend to give birth. Your partner will no doubt want to play an active part during the birth of your child, and he can begin to do this by safeguarding your integrity during your preparation time. This too is part of childbirth. Do not to allow it to become a hyperintended process.

Your partner can also help by looking after your other children, taking calls, finding his favourite black sweater himself etc. You are preparing to give birth consciously; what you are doing is truly important. Do the following exercise daily, from six months through pregnancy or earlier.

Deep relaxation exercise

Sit comfortably, remove watches and anything that will make you uncomfortable during the next half hour.

Let go of the future. It will all be there waiting for you when you get back. You can safely let it go for this short time. Let go of the past. Leave it all behind for now. This is the moment when you can begin to repair the past and prepare the future. Be here, now, to do your exercise with all your attention, fully in this moment.

Relax your crown. You can imagine warm treacle pouring down your crown and over your head and face.
Relax your forehead.
Relax your eyebrows. Relax the area between your eyebrows.
Relax all the fine muscles around your eyes.
Relax your cheeks.
Your lips.
Your jaw.
Relax the back of your head, your scalp.
Relax your neck.
Relax your throat.

Relax your left arm, letting the tension pour out, down the arm, starting with your shoulder, down through your upper arm, your elbow, your lower arm, your wrist, your hand and out through each one of the fingers.

Relax your right arm, letting the tension pour out, down the arm, starting with your shoulder, down through your upper arm, your elbow, your lower arm, your wrist, your hand and out through each one of the fingers.

Relax your chest.
Relax your upper back.

Relax your abdomen, which can hold so much tension.
Relax your lower back.

Relax the sex function and the pelvic area. The womb, vagina, labia, inside of the thighs, the anus, buttocks. This is the area that will soon work beautifully for you and you need to get to know it well.

Relax your left leg, starting from the hip and feeling the tension moving out through the thigh, the knee, the calf, the ankle, the foot and out through each one of the toes.

Relax your right leg, starting from the hip and feeling the tension moving out through the thigh, the knee, the calf, the ankle, the foot and out through each one of the toes.

Sense your right foot, feel sensation creeping in, from the toes and filling the whole of the foot. Let the sensation of your living body fill your calf, rising up through the thigh and up to the hip. Fill with sensation.

Let sensation flow in through your left foot, from the toes and rising up, filling the left leg to the hip.

Let sensation enter your pelvis, sense your internal organs working for you. Sense your labia, vagina, womb, your thighs, buttocks, anus.

Feel sensation filling you, moving up your lower back, filling your abdomen.

Feel sensation rising through your chest, filling your upper back.

Fill your neck and throat with sensation.

Be aware of your spine, your axis, your central pole.

Feel sensation fill the muscles of your face, your head, your scalp, all the way up to the crown.

Be aware of your body, your organism as a whole. Take some time to just be in this state. When you notice your thoughts starting to wander, return back to sensation. Stay with the sensation of your living body.

Be aware when you leave the exercise; know that you are now going back into your usual life. Start moving your fingers and toes and gradually come back to the room around you.

Learn to do this exercise by heart so that you can do it sitting still, with your eyes closed. Do it daily, in the morning. It will bring you in closer contact with your tissues and organs, with your physical body, and help you better understand your role during childbirth.

Preparing for labour

When you know the exercise well, start to do it in labouring positions. We do not know in advance what these will be, but experiment and find out what you feel most comfortable with. You may find that the positions that you find most comfortable are different for each birth.

Try sitting on a chair, leaning forward onto your folded arms supported by a desk. Keep your eyes closed. Let your attention go inward.

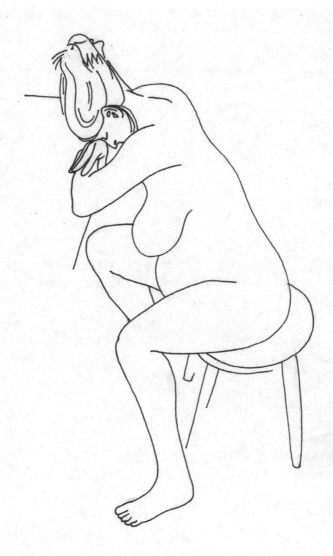

Try standing up, supported on either side by something firm and stable such as two bookshelves, hanging onto them with both arms, almost dangling. Try hanging on your partner, with your arms around his neck.

Try leaning forward on a beanbag or large cushion on the floor, kneeling and clasping around the cushion with your arms.

Try kneeling at the end of the bed with your upper body and arms stretched out in front of you.

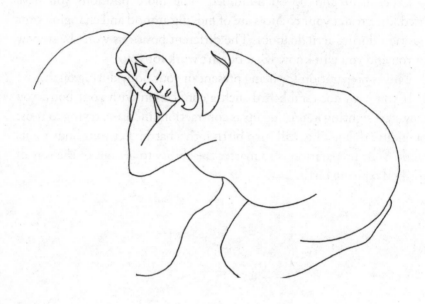

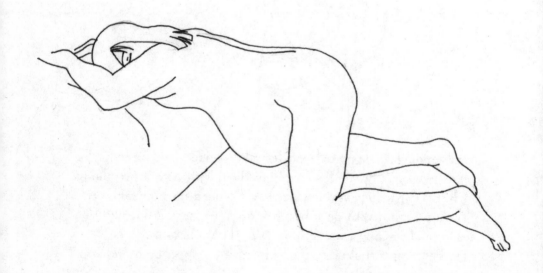

Try lying down on a bed or sofa with one leg raised so that your knee is against your chest.

Experiment and be open-minded. The more positions you have tried, the greater your chances are of moving around and changing your position during actual labour. The different positions won't be so new to you and you will know what doesn't work for you.

This is preparation for being present in your body during birth.

If you have not established such a connection with your body, you may start fighting it, tensing up as contractions increase, trying to resist or endure them. This will turn birth into a battle. Let your body do its work. Your preparation is to master the ability to get out of the way of the body during birth.

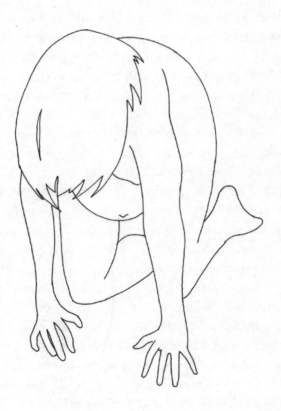

Communicating with your tissues

When you have established this connection through regular exercises, you can 'visit' areas that you wish to know more about. Do the deep relaxation exercise fully. Maintain that state. Now go to the area closest to the point you wish to 'visit' which is on the outside of your body. For example, if you wish to visit your womb, sense your labia. Sense them as fully as you can, then move up through the vagina, again sensing the tissues fully. Continue to move up into the womb, all the time sensing the tissues. You may now be able to make a connection and increase your awareness of what is happening in your womb. You could also start from your belly button and move inwards through layers of tissue. The important thing is to keep sensation constant.

A wise person once said that if you have dropped a glass and it's lying on the floor smashed into a thousand fragments, all you can do is to accept that it is so — the glass has already been smashed — and to move on from there. If a glass is balancing precariously at the edge of a table and may fall, it is still possible to nudge it further onto the table so that the risk of falling is eliminated. Finally, if a glass is already in midair, falling and on its way to the floor, it is still possible to catch it and return it to the table intact. In a similar way, it may be possible for you to see a problem and resolve it before it actually becomes manifest in a physical symptom.

There are many documented incidences of how the mind can influence the workings of the physical body in a positive way, so this is not just an exercise in imagination. You can use your imagination in a directed manner to connect with the part of you that is usually hidden, your instinctive function.

I had four miscarriages before and between successful pregnancies. When eighteen weeks pregnant with my daughter I started bleeding and having menstrual-type contractions. I carried out the exercise of connecting with my tissues and was able to tell that the glass had not yet fallen, and I was able to put it firmly on the table. It is possible to influence early contractions through meditation, deep relaxation exercises or self-hypnosis. If in doubt, get help.

However, here is another warning: be wary of imagination. It may mislead you. There is no foolproof way. Yet it is still possible to deepen your understanding and awareness of your body, and even to communicate with your instinctive parts. Communication between 'you' and functions or organs within you may take the form of dreams, or images flashing by, visions, even voices or thoughts appearing in your mind out of 'nowhere.' But first it is necessary to become aware of all the junk that usually floats around our minds, so that we can distinguish between genuine communications from our instinctive function and mere imagination.

In such a deeply relaxed state as described above it is possible to communicate with the foetus. Hold the state and be open. You cannot force it. It is possible for your children to name themselves. This cannot be verified by anyone but yourself in relation to your child. No one can ever scientifically verify that you love your partner. Yet it is true. Empirical study is not the only way of ascertaining truths.

When you are familiar with the deep relaxation exercise, use a birthing CD. There are several good CDs available. Dr Gowri Motha's *The Jeyarani Way* is particularly helpful as it focuses on anatomical detail and processes during labour. There will be others that work for you (see Resources). Associating the birthing process with this deeply relaxed state will help make your birth easier.

Continue to work on sensing your body — individual parts, organs, your womb, vagina, labia, pelvic floor etc. Study anatomy and physiology in order to know and be able to sense your body more fully, to establish a clearer connection with your tissues and functions. We live so much in our heads that we are unaware of many of our functions and do not sense our tissues as we should or can.

Begin to listen to self-hypnosis CDs as early as possible during pregnancy. This will allow your body time to adjust to the messages you wish it to take in and for you to become more aware of the process unfolding within you. It will also give you time to work on your subconscious attitudes to childbirth. Give your body and yourself plenty of time to prepare for this awe-inspiring experience.

It is a momentous thing. A new being is coming in to the three-dimensional world of space and time. A new and completely unique aspect of the Absolute is being born. And you are the instrument. Childbirth enables the possibility of a connection with spiritual truth, or that truth which lies beyond body. Your body is the vehicle that enables a miraculous process to take place. Higher forces pass through you and woman becomes the agent of the higher. This begins with sensing your body.

Preparing visual material

Collecting and preparing visual material to be used as an aid to the birthing woman can be very helpful. It is also a way of communicating with your partner during birth. Words may be hard to get out as all your resources become focused on the tissues around your womb and birthing canal. It is literally difficult to speak, and even to hear. Spend some time thinking about which images you associate with smooth, gradual opening and release. Such images might include rose buds opening, a diaphragm spreading outwards or a camera aperture fanning out. Use your imagination!

Carefully choose images which have the most positive and gentle associations for you and include this library of images in your birth preparation. Note down the words that best express what will be happening to your cervix. Unfurling, unwinding, separating, spreading, thinning might be amongst the words that have the best effect on you. Keep them locked away in the secret chambers of your psyche. They will come to you when you most need them.

Continue to practise sensing the tissues of your cervix. From 38 weeks, in your daily exercise, you can include sensing your cervical tissues while visualizing flowers unfurling, opening, separating. You can prepare the ground for the actual birth, meaning that a large part of the work will already have been done when the day comes. If you carry out these exercises, you may find that your mucal plug will be released during these last two weeks, without necessarily heralding the imminent birth of your child.

Warning: do not visualize these images or intone these words while sensing your cervix until it is time, no earlier than 38 weeks. The effect is real and could trigger premature birth.

As your contractions intensify, it may be helpful if your partner shows you these images, presents them to you, and you can delve into them visually as you dive into the great ocean beyond time. Don't worry if you end up pushing them away with an expletive on the day. It doesn't matter: the preparation will not be wasted and will be used by some other part of your psyche. Prepare thoroughly, but be ready to abandon your plan at any minute in order to be fully in the present, responding to the reality as it is, not as you might have wished it to be.

Hold on tightly, let go lightly.

Preparing temperature, light and sound

You need to be able to easily regulate the temperature of the room in which you intend to give birth. The birthing mother may need a relatively warm room to start with when she is more still and quiet, and then later, as contractions increase and this great physical work heats up her body and brings sweat to her brow, she will probably want a cooler room. This may sound obvious, but trying to sort it out on the day, in the midst of overwhelming physical and emotional experiences and lots of other seriously pressing needs, could become farcical and traumatic quite quickly.

If you feel that listening to music would help you during your birth, choose meditative, tranquil, calm music as you will probably not be aware of hearing much of it on the day, but it will go straight into your subconscious mind. Skip anything with negative lyrics or too fast a beat as this will influence you subtly too. Aim to keep yourself calm, meditative, focused and joyful.

Try to keep the lighting low, as your newborn baby will soon be experiencing light entering her eye for the very first time, and because it will enhance your meditative, inward-looking state.

Preparing other people — children

Make sure there is no one present at your birth who might make you feel restrained or inhibited. If there are unresolved issues between you and your birthing partner or anyone else who is going to be present during the birth, aim to resolve these by eight weeks before the birth. If they cannot be resolved, work to accept this and do not allow them to be present during the birth. Otherwise, the tension will hinder the smooth flow of energies through your tissues.

If other children are present, ensure that the mother is always put first, do not allow them to distract her. If you feel you cannot ensure this through the help of your birthing partner, do not allow children to be present. Take responsibility for your birth. Your children have the natural ability to suck every ounce of your resources towards them and are, as they are not yet mature, quite selfish. You will not be able to firmly tell them that Mummy needs to be undisturbed, or needs peace and quiet, or can't help them right now without expending a considerable amount of energy. And an exceptional amount of energy is required to give birth. Do not spend it lightly.

Preparing yourself for birth

It takes about the same amount of energy to give birth as it does to run a marathon.

In the weeks immediately before birth, the mother needs to get as much sleep as she can. She needs to be rested when labour begins, so forget all the commitments you can, just catnap and rest whenever you are able to. Sleep at night will probably be quite shallow because of the weight of the foetus and other discomforts such as pressure on your bladder, so make sure that you nap as often as possible.

Start eating endurance foods at around 38 weeks in preparation for birth; you never know which will be your last meal before labour begins! You probably won't be able to eat large quantities as your stomach will be squeezed by the foetus, but try to eat often. Include pasta, oats, fruit, nuts and yoghurt as these will give you the long-lasting energy reserves you will need during labour.

Addressing fears

The first thing is: they are not yours.

If fears regarding birth appear in your mind, draw them, write them down, capture them. Otherwise they slip away and hide in the recesses of your mind and cannot be neutralized by the light of day and the power of your rational mind, which will see their fantasist imagination running riot. Bring your fears into the light. Don't let them tyrannize your subconscious world.

In your relaxed state, visualize your birth. How do you wish it to be? See it progress before your inner eye. See the result, the outcome on the other side of the momentous experience you are privilege to. Try to do this daily for the last ten weeks of pregnancy.

Working to visualize how you would like your birth to be will help, because we attract our reality by our (conscious or subconscious) expectations.

See yourself after the birth, holding your baby. Imagination is a powerful tool if used in a *controlled* way, instead of wasting our energies in daydreaming or negative fantasies about everything that might go wrong in our life — *uncontrolled* imagination. It needs to be directed to be of service to you.

Actively use your imagination to make this image of you cradling your baby a fact. It has already happened in eternity. It is already a reality. You know the future and all you need to do now is to walk the way there, to go through the motions. You need to go through the transformative trial of childbirth, to act out your part, here, in space and time.

Connecting with the fourth dimension

The perceptions possible for any being are limited by the number of dimensions of the world she inhabits. However, she may be able to develop in herself functions that can begin to access a higher dimension. This is the real, psychological meaning of religion, of all the great religions: re-establishing the connection, the link, with a higher dimension.

Re-ligion: from *re* = *again*, *ligare* = *bind*. Religion is, or should be, a linking again, back to the place or state from whence we have come, re-connecting with the higher. Re-membering ourselves, like Osiris in Egyptian myth, who was first torn asunder, limb from limb, to then be re-membered and rise again.

So from this perspective, the fourth dimension is a kind of new direction in relation to us. It is not height, width or length. It is something hitherto unknown to us.

The geometry of the fourth dimension

Mathematically, dimension refers to the number of co-ordinates needed to describe a point. The world of zero dimension can be represented by a point. It has no width, length or height and is infinitely small.

The world of one dimension can be represented by a line and is accessed by making a vertical projection away from the world of no dimension, the world of the point. A line has one dimension — length. The width and height of a line are infinitely small. Each part of the line is comprised of a zero-dimensional object — a point. An infinite line would cover all of one-dimensional space.

The world of two dimensions can be represented by a triangle and is accessed by making a vertical projection away from the world of one dimension, the world of the line. A triangle has two dimensions — length and width. The height of a two-dimensional object is infinitely small. Each side of the triangle is comprised of a one-dimensional object — a line. If you expand the triangle infinitely it would cover all of two-dimensional space.

The world of three dimensions can be represented by a tetrahedron and is accessed by making a vertical projection away from the world of two dimensions, the world of the plane. A tetrahedron has three dimensions — length, width and height. Each side of the tetrahedron is comprised of a two-dimensional object — a triangle. If you expand the tetrahedron infinitely it would cover all of three-dimensional space. We live and move in three-dimensional space, the world of space and time.

If we imagine, then, that the fourth dimension is extended similarly in a perpendicular fashion away from three-dimensional space, it would be extended out of space and time. The fourth dimension lies beyond the world that we can perceive with our senses.

One way to understand four dimensions is to look closely at how we can understand three dimensions using only images drawn in the plane. How we use these two-dimensional images to reconstruct in our heads the full three-dimensional objects can serve as a basis for trying to use three-dimensional pictures to construct four-dimensional objects in our heads in a similar way. We can use our imagination to visualize that each side of a four-dimensional object would be comprised of a three-dimensional object.

The addition of another dimension brings with it many possibilities that do not exist in the dimension below it. For example, a two-dimensional being has the possibility of movement in two directions, where a one-dimensional being can only move along the line which constitutes its dimension. However, a two-dimensional being can only see what lies in its plane of existence. A three-dimensional being has many possibilities not open to a two-dimensional being. It can move upwards into the dimension of height. A three-dimensional being moving through a two-dimensional world would appear 'super-natural,' could perform 'miracles.'

It may be said that birth actually begins around eight weeks before labour. You may experience a gradual retreat into your self, into your instinctive parts. Habits that lie in personality are weakened and you may find yourself becoming more simple, more immediate. You begin to live more in essence and function and less in personality. You may find yourself less able to play the games of social interaction.

So at 32 weeks, allow your labour to begin, slowly, softly. Allow personality to withdraw and retreat, allow yourself to sink deeper and deeper into your true self. Wind down your commitments. Don't make yourself talk to people if you feel uncommunicative. Give yourself permission to be fully in this experience of slowing down your outer life so that you may fully go to the place where the outer can connect with the inner — the place where the third dimension can connect with the fourth.

You have the possibility of delving into the mysteries of woman, to reach the place where birth and death meet and complete the cycle through you, through an already existing female body. This is the connecting point in eternity. The child's first gasp of air is the last breath drawn by the dying man at the end of his cycle. He goes out of space and time and enters eternity, while instantly, in space and time, he is born again.

> *In my beginning is my end ...*
> *In my end is my beginning.*
> (From 'East Coker,' *Four Quartets*, T.S. Eliot)

As woman, you have the great privilege of being invited to become an initiate of the mysteries beyond time. You may enter the hall of eternity through your conscious obeisance to the forces of nature, of organic life on earth, and those that lie beyond, in the fourth dimension, or the realm of spirit.

5. Childbirth

What happens before birth?

In the weeks before birth, hormones are secreted that allow your muscles and tissues to soften. However, this in no way compromises their strength. The placenta secretes the pregnancy hormone relaxin, which helps your joints and bones become flexible. The genetic make-up that you have inherited from your ancestors means that when your baby is born, she will be the perfect size to pass through your pelvis and birth canal. In the last few weeks of pregnancy, your baby naturally settles into the ideal position for birth, which is head down, with the spine facing outwards. This is known as the anterior position.

At 38 weeks, your cervix begins to thin and soften and stretch in readiness for birth. Vizualization can help the cervix to open bit by bit every day, making the day of the birth itself easier.

In the weeks before birth, your cervix also releases a smooth mucus in preparation for your baby's passage down the birth canal. Day by day, your baby sinks down, settling deeper and deeper into the uterus; your midwife may call this 'being engaged.' You can encourage your baby to settle into the anterior position by tilting you pelvis forward, i.e. sitting with your knees lower than your back or resting on all fours. You will notice that your baby starts to move less, as there is not much room and because she sinks into herself, in preparation for entering fully into the world of space and time.

Your baby still remembers why she is coming into the world and joyfully anticipates being held in your arms. She knows the value of the gift of life that you are making possible for her in a way that we can only strive to understand later in life. To honour your mother and your father, to be fully aware of what your parents have truly done for you, including at a biological level, is a high level of being. Your baby comes into this world full of gratitude.

When your baby has completed all her growth processes and is truly ready to come into the world, many scientists now believe that she triggers the release of prostaglandins, which instruct your body to begin the process of birthing; your baby chooses the moment of birth herself. Once these messages have reached your brain, they trigger the release of oxytocin, which causes your womb to contract — very gently at first, gradually gathering momentum.

The prospect of the birth drawing closer may seem frightening. Keep dealing with any residual fears by confronting them and putting them down on paper. Keep revealing them to the light of day; expose them to your rational mind. This is a most precious opportunity to experience the awesome power and complexity of your body, what it really is and what it can do. It is well known that we use only a fraction of our brain's real capacity. It is also true that we use only a fraction of our physical possibilities. The body is mind-bogglingly sophisticated, powerful and wondrous. During birth, it is possible to catch a glimpse of the extent of the miracle that the life force performs through matter every minute of every day.

During birth, your uterus and pelvis will gradually and gently open up. This can take a number of hours or maybe days. Allow it to take its time. Remember that your baby is coming because she wishes to with all her being, that she herself has initiated the birth process and that she has chosen you as her mother. She is waiting patiently to see you. It is possible to reciprocate this expectation and acceptance.

The anatomy of your pelvis and womb

The pelvis is composed of four inter-connected bones: the two hip bones and the sacrum and the coccyx at the back. It is through the opening between these bones that your baby will pass. When your baby's head presses against the pelvic bones, they shift and flex to allow your baby to slide through. Your baby's head is also soft and flexible, allowing it to adapt to the size of your pelvis and birth canal.

The perineum is a stretchy muscle that lines the opening of the pelvis. This strong muscle gently holds and protects your womb. Fat and connective tissue also cushion the pelvis at the top and bottom of the perineum. There is plenty of space for a baby to pass through and there are many layers of soft tissue that are designed to yield as your baby moves down the birth canal.

Your womb is made up of long and very strong muscle fibres. These are layered and interwoven to maximize strength.

The tissues in your vagina are composed of elastic fibres that stretch and rebound with surprising ease. The slippery mucus membranes that line your vagina consist of fold upon fold of tissue that will fan out and open wide when it is time for your baby to pass through.

The intelligence of your instinctive function knows exactly what to do, and is able to open up a safe passage to let your baby enter the world. After birth, your tissues quickly and easily return to their usual size and your womb returns back to a state of quiet preparedness.

The physiological process of birth

Specialized nerve endings called stretch receptors are located throughout the body to communicate changes in tone, volume and tension. Once your child has started the birthing process, the stretch receptors located in the lower uterus and cervix send a message to your pituitary gland to release more oxytocin. The oxytocin is then carried in the blood back to the womb, where it causes the uterus to contract. The contracting uterus then activates the stretch receptors to send more neurological signals to the brain, which stimulates more oxytocin release, leading to the longer duration and closer frequency of contractions. The birth of your child eventually terminates this sequence.

During birth, the strong, interwoven muscle tissues that are your womb contract from the top down. Each contraction puts firm, downward pressure onto your baby. The force generated by the womb passes through the baby's body and pushes the baby's head against the cervix, activating the stretch receptors. The cervix opens gradually, like a camera lens.

Every time the uterus contracts, the cervix is pulled open a little further by special fibres that connect it to the womb. After a number of contractions, the cervix will be fully dilated, allowing your baby's head access to the full vaginal space. During the next contraction, your baby's head begins to pass down through your vagina. Each ensuing contraction gradually pushes the baby further down the vagina. You will start to feel a great, irresistible urge to push yourself, and you will soon push your baby out through the vaginal opening and into the world.

The more deeply you are able to relax during birth, the more energy you will have for use during labour. This energy can then be used specifically by your womb, allowing it to do its work unimpaired. Complete relaxation allows your automatic muscles to work unhindered. The systems that need to work during childbirth are your breathing, your heartbeat and the contractions of your womb. Complete relaxation means that no energy is wasted on unnecessary tension and that those parts of you that are working can carry out their task with ease.

Birth itself

When contractions begin, relax in the space you have prepared for giving birth. Turn down the light and make sure you are undisturbed. Put on some music or just relax into the workings of your wonderful body. You will find that your contractions gradually become more powerful.

If you stay clear of the temptations of drugs and birth by elective caesarean, you will experience a gradual altering of your state of consciousness. Endorphins (the word comes from *endogenous morphine*, i.e. morphine produced by your own body) are released in your body when you experience pain, when you exercise or relax deeply, as well as when you feel comfort, pleasure or enthusiasm. As you give birth to your child, your body releases endorphins to give you natural pain relief and help you to relax. You can then gradually turn more and more inwards until the outside world begins to seem less real than your inner world.

Submitting to the gradual release of endorphins keeps you relaxed and focussed. The steady supply of endorphins generated by each contraction ensures that you always have the right amount in your bloodstream. Allow yourself to sink into the rhythm of the coming and going of the contractions, let the sea of contractions wash over you. Go along with the push and pull of each wave. There is a long rest between each contraction; use it to sink deeper and deeper into relaxation and allow your partner to replenish your resources.

You have prepared carefully for this birth and you can now reap the benefits of all your efforts. The exercises you have been practising will allow you to easily fall into a state of deep relaxation, and even to fall asleep, between each contraction.

> Helpful words and images: slip, wet, stretch, thin, out, easy,
> beautiful, safe, comfortable, soft, mouldable, loving, kind.

Remember that your baby is as prepared as you are, having benefited from sharing in your state during your deep relaxation exercises.

All your birthing tissues come into their own at this moment. Your body is serving you lovingly, focussing all its resources on ensuring the safe birth of your child. Only a few times in your life will your wonderful womb be able to show what it is truly capable of, and today is the day.

You sink deeper and deeper into a hypnotic state of profound relaxation. When the next contraction comes along you relax deep into it and pass through it entirely relaxed, allowing only the automatic muscle functioning of your instinctive parts. The more you relax, the easier it is to produce oxytocin.

You let go of the room around you and delve deep into yourself to the place where your glorious body functions entirely unhindered.

Your calm, deep breathing in the quiet periods between contractions allows you to send more oxygen to your bloodstream, benefiting both you and your baby. Steadily take small amounts of food and liquid, as this sends glucose from your liver to your womb, so that you and your baby are always well prepared for the next contraction.

You have to go somewhere else to give birth. Between contractions, which take you over entirely, you do not merely return to your usual state, where you might ask what time it is or wonder how someone else is doing. During and also between contractions, you go to a relaxed, much deeper state, closer to your true self, where time and place do not exist.

As your baby travels down the birth canal, you start to feel your baby's head in the lower part of your vagina. It feels like a fullness and you may feel like you want to open your bowel. This means that your child is now about to come into the world. Keep breathing deeply and relax into this sensation. It is healthy and normal to want to empty your bowel during childbirth; do not hold back. Also remember that there is evidence that it is beneficial for a baby to come into contact with its mother's faecal matter during birth, as it can protect your baby from developing allergies later in life.

Lying down on your left side is known to help labour to progress more quickly, should you need it.

Your body continues to send out large quantities of endorphins, giving you a natural high, and continuously reigns in any sensation of pain. The endorphins help you feel calm and blissful during and between contractions. Allow yourself to enjoy the endorphins and let them help you to relax deeper and deeper into the place where you can fully give yourself over to your body. Here, you let go of the 'control' you believe you have in ordinary life. You see that what exercises this control is in fact not you, just a small part of you. Giving yourself up shows you what you truly are and what you might become.

Keep breathing in deep relaxation and visualize the muscles of your vagina unfolding and opening out. As your baby's head begins to appear at the opening of your vagina you will be overcome with an overwhelming feeling that you are right here, right now more than you ever have been before. You feel an incredible bursting sensation and a wonderful, ecstatic experience all at once. You can reach down and touch your baby's wet hair. It is really happening now: you are really here, in the most incredible moment of all existence. Your baby is coming.

The next contraction requires only a little push from you to assist it.

Once the baby's head is born, you experience a wonderful feeling of release and all is very easy after that. The rest of your baby slips through like a wet seal. Your placenta will soon follow at its own pace.

The advantage of taking responsibility for your own birth, whether you call it a home birth, a natural birth or a conscious birth, is that this will allow you to be more present at your births. You may experience unbearable pain, and yet you will bear it. This is what allows you to become Mother. You were there, present during your child's birth. You were not running away from pain, from fear, from expectations. You were there. You assumed responsibility for your birth and you stood firm.

You may receive your child with your own hands, feel her wet crown crowning, hold her head as it passes through, cradle her shoulders, firmly grip her slippery arm, hold her in your two hands and lift her to your breast. You give birth to your child. You need not be a passive participant in a process of which you understand little. You can be the instrument of the birth of your child. You can be there, you can feel the pain, you can stand up to it and take your child from your womb like the woman you have become.

What happens after birth

After the birth, your baby continues to receive oxygen from the placenta for a while, even after she has begun breathing independently. You can see the umbilical cord continuing to pulsate and you may want to wait to cut the cord until this has stopped. This also means that your baby will continue to share your endorphins for a time after being born and you will both feel euphoric and alert.

When the placenta senses that your baby is breathing independently and regularly, it sends a message to your womb, making it contract firmly. These last few contractions allow you to easily push the placenta out through the vagina. The magnificent placenta has now completed its complex and difficult task and is no longer needed. Now is an opportunity to admire its beauty and allow yourself to feel the respect it deserves. The midwife will carefully examine it to ensure that it is intact. If part of the placenta remains in the womb it can cause infection and it will need to be removed. After the placenta has been expelled, your uterus remains firmly contracted, ensuring that there is only slight bleeding. Some parents bury the placenta and plant a tree for the child over it.

You will gradually return to the shape you had before you became pregnant, only now you will be even more beautiful because you have become a Mother who knows.

The first breath

Your adrenaline levels are never higher than while you are being born. Adrenaline boosts the oxygen supply and helps prepare the lungs to breathe. Adrenaline also increases blood pressure, heart rate, the volume of blood being pumped around your body and releases glucose from the liver, which raises blood sugar levels. The foetus' adrenal glands secrete large quantities of adrenaline and noradrenaline during birth. These hormones protect the foetus from oxygen starvation during the powerful contractions that squeeze not only the baby but also the umbilical cord. Adrenaline also prepares the lungs for taking their first breath by reducing the formation of lung fluid and widening the respiratory tracts.

When your baby takes its first breath, 25 million alveoli are filled with air for the first time. They will contain lung fluid initially, although this is quickly dispersed into the bloodstream and lymphatic system. In a moment, the entire circulatory system of your baby is rearranged. The hole in the wall between the atria of the heart closes, never to be opened again, and the baby immediately begins to rely on its own independent supply of oxygen.

The newborn baby's first breath gives the signal to all vital life systems to start working independently. In an instant, a complete and mind-bogglingly complex system comes into full flow. It has had no trial runs, no real-time tests. Air begins to be included and transformed in countless processes in the human body. The shock of air puts the seal on life. It is a shock that will be maintained through life, at every breath drawn, allowing the body to burn the food that is taken into the digestive tract and transform it into finer energies, such as movement, thought, feeling. There is no turning back now.

I am alive. I have a body and have fully entered the world with my first breath. I am.

Time is breath. Time begins with breath. Upon your first breath, time begins to count for you.

The moment of birth — bonding

The first prolonged eye contact is magical. This is the moment of connection and recognition of each other, the mother and child in the roles that they are set to play for the lifetime ahead. It is not generally acknowledged as such. The newborn knows, she has not yet forgotten. We are set to dance this beautiful dance; you are mother, I am child. Do you remember?

As you gaze into the mysteriously coloured eyes of your newborn, you may find yourself falling in love. It is as deep and overwhelming as when you fall in love with your future partner. The strength of emotion can be surprisingly sudden. Most babies are alert during their first few hours after birth, and later sleep deeply for several hours. Make the most of this first, precious time.

Close observation and eye contact, breastfeeding and being held and warmed all contribute to the building of emotional function. The baby continues to share in your hormonal secretions through breast milk, and you maintain the sharing of emotions outside the womb by keeping the child in close proximity, in your cloud of hormones, in the radiance of love. The child shares in all the other workings, positive or negative, of the mother's emotional function, and so we learn what emotions should feel like.

Emotional function, when working correctly, is the source of love, hope and faith, and can develop its own intelligence. Likes and dislikes, which rightly belong to instinctive function, creep in to emotional function during childhood. We become hypnotized that we have a right to anger, irritation and self-pity, when joy, love and peace are our birthright. Instinctive function counts only to two: it divides impressions entering the organism through the senses into pain/ pleasure, hot/cold, rough/smooth. We learn through imitation that when something hurts, which is a sensation, we should also *feel* bad.

The way you look at your newborn child is with a degree of attention, an emotional and physical presence that is rarely reproduced. You will be more attentive that any machine or doctor and can read your child's feelings and needs on her face, in her movements and in her voice. You are the best-equipped person in the world to do this, by virtue of being the child's mother. This is increasingly recognized by medical professionals and it has been found to be more expedient to listen to the mother's 'intuition' or 'instinct' than to rely exclusively on tests and examinations.

It is possible to observe in yourself a very special kind of affinity with your newborn child. Sometimes you may sense what they are sensing; it is as if pain or sensation becomes transferred, very lightly, but nevertheless perceptibly. It is possible to experience in your body what your child is experiencing. This continues for a few years after birth, to be increasingly supplanted by the use of language as the child grows older.

6. Spiritual Birth

Conscious labour

What does it mean to do something consciously? It is something that we do *with intention* and through the fullness of the faculties available to us here in three-dimensional space. If we *repair* and *prepare* the faculties we have in this world of senses, they may become perfected enough to just touch the higher faculties that have lain beyond our reach up until now. If we make effort from below, it is met with help from above. Artists, mystics, poets and wise men and women speak of such a possibility.

Time as we usually perceive it is an illusion, and woman is blessed with the ability to experience the real forces of the universe that act beyond this veil of matter that we call our lives. Preparation for this moment allows her to savour as much of it as possible, placing within her reach the moment where linear time intersects with eternity.

We may then tap into what is rightfully ours. It might be called a higher state of consciousness. Some call it cosmic consciousness. Others call it revelation, mystical states, visions, ah-ha moments, a moment when time stands still. So, by repairing and capitalizing on what we have been given, we may receive more. The striving towards consciousness is transformative.

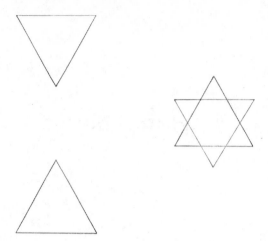

My effort from below to complete that which is not whole is met with help from above. This is the true meaning of prayer.

On our way through life, learning through the experiences our life so generously provides, we have the potential to transform that part of us which lies beyond the material body. To become aware of this possibility is our first task. We may then encounter a guide on the way and come to realize that it is for precisely this reason that we have chosen to come here: to transform ourselves.

Consciousness may sound like something that you already possess, or like a very high and mysterious concept. Like charity, it begins at home. What is your being? What are you? Not your job, not your name, not your past, but the sum total of your everyday actions. How do you manifest? Do you know yourself? Do you know how others see you? Not as you think they see you. Not as you would like them to see you. How do you actually appear? You cannot see yourself from outside. Through intentional, directed work and through sharing experiences with others it is possible to allow others to act as a mirror. You may then be able to see yourself from outside for a moment and come to know how you actually are. Your tone of voice, your gestures, your choice of words, what your eyes do and don't reveal about your inner state, your moods, your posture — all this is largely hidden from us, even though it is blindingly obvious to those around us. Peering out through our

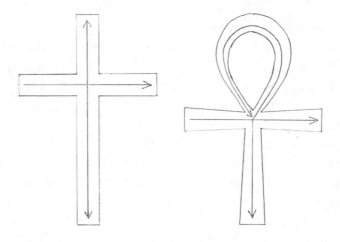

Many ancient symbols contain a great deal of information that we can apply to our lives if we can learn how to read them. The symbol of the cross is pervasive and not limited to Christianity, while the Ankh symbol is central to the ancient Egyptian culture and incorporates many levels of meaning. 'Chronos' is ancient Greek for time and Chronos time expresses linear time as we usually perceive it, symbolized by the horizontal part of both the cross and the Ankh. 'Kairos' is ancient Greek for the supreme moment, which we usually only experience at peak moments in our life — moments when time stops, or becomes elastic. It is our point of connection with eternity, time out of time. Kairos time intersects Chronos time in both the symbol of the cross and the Ankh. The potential to connect with eternity is present in every moment. In the Ankh, Kairos time is shown as returning back down to Chronos time, revealing the possibility of eternal recurrence.

eyes we assume that the world can sense our real motives and that we can hide our feelings when we wish to. This is not so. We cannot. The ancient Greek aphorism that was inscribed in the Temple of Apollo at Delphi, 'Know thyself,' is only the first rung of the ladder towards self-perfection, towards building something imperishable and objective, towards building a soul.

Your being may be anchored in your education. By educating yourself you change your being slightly. You become a little different. You begin to manifest a little differently as a result of new things that you have learned.

Conscious labour is about not just letting it happen. If we were normal women, as we were intended to be, we could perhaps just let it happen; if our instinctive function were allowed to do its job without interference from our misaligned psyche or from contemporary medicine, that is. In the world in which we live, everything just happens, and everything follows the path of least resistance. It may certainly seem as though you fight against resistance in your life, but in fact we all follow the path of least resistance *for ourselves*. For example, if I have a firmly embedded notion in my psyche that I am terrible at maths, I will go through life avoiding jobs that require maths, avoiding getting involved in splitting the bill in restaurants and so on. This is the path of least resistance for me, although it may seem as if I spend my life struggling with maths. To not follow the path of least resistance would be to become aware of the voice at the back of my mind that keeps telling me that I'm no good at maths and to challenge it.

If we do not become aware of what we are, of these subconscious behaviours and inner attitudes, we continue to encounter the particular sufferings to which we are prone. 'I'm bad at maths' or 'I'm just too scared of something going wrong to consider home birth' becomes a self-fulfilling prophecy and my possibility of living life to the full is limited by it.

Like most of life, birth too can just happen. Then it will be the result of your subconscious expectations and the expectations of those around you. Conscious labour is the result of preparation and the intentional accumulation of knowledge and being that allows the potentially transformative experience of birth to reach its highest potential. You are invited, as the representative of woman, to partake in the mysteries that lie beyond time.

Don't let your birth just happen, don't allow it to be pushed along by expectations — your own subconscious expectations, foisted on you by your education, upbringing and conditioning, or the expectations of those around you: 'But don't most people give birth in hospital?' 'Aren't you scared of not having doctors at hand?' 'What if something goes wrong?' 'Don't you think you would be safer in hospital?' 'The best procedures have been put in place by the people that know best, the experts.' You may be tempted to compromise, to go to hospital after all, even though you would have liked to give birth at home, for example. You may not sufficiently trust your intuition about giving birth, and there is only little support to be found for going against the grain. Governed by fear, your universe will soon become a small prison indeed.

Research birth. Find out as much as you can about the stages of labour. Read about home births. Read about hospital procedures. Read about the psychology of pregnancy and childbirth, about the effect hormones have on a woman's mind and body. Make the birth yours. Don't just let it happen. This is a step towards a higher level of consciousness. By becoming an active participant rather than a passive leaf floating along on the eddies and currents of life you are changing your being, the sum total of what you are, all your manifestations combined. Make your birth conscious.

Bring what you are expecting (that which has been hidden in your subconscious until now) to the surface. Look at it. Examine it with your intellect. Let the light of day shine on it. Fairy tales teach us that a troll cannot survive the light of day. Let the light of day shine into the hidden world of your subconscious expectations. Let your consciousness expose the trolls lurking in the darkness. Become aware of your subconscious expectations. Make them conscious.

From God to man

One.
In the beginning was the Word and the Word was with God and the Word was God. This is the source of all things existing, the unmanifest thought that lies at the core of all creation. It is the Word because it has not become manifest, it has no matter, it is purely thought, idea, Word. The Absolute. Alpha and Omega. All and Everything. Eternity. Infinity. The Whole.
One.

Two.
God beholds himself, becomes self-aware. In Egyptian creation

myth, Tum beholds himself and begets Atum. Through becoming aware of yourself, by separating yourself inwardly so that one part is as before and one part observes, you can become Two. One passes into Two.
Two.

Three.
Two gives birth to a shared understanding, the space between two overlapping circles, the Vesica Pisces from which all numbers spring. The birth of Three: that which You can understand only by Yourself and for Yourself, the first circle, and that which I can understand only by Myself and for Myself, the second circle, and that which We can understand Together, the Vesica Pisces. This raises the understanding of both to a new level.
Three.

Four.
The abstract idea of Three can become manifest in the physical world of three dimensions, in space and time, and take on form, a body. Three becomes Four, allowing the Word to become manifest. Four points of the compass. Four legs of a table. Four sides of a square. Four denotes stability, earth, matter. When a woman becomes a mother, Mater, she acts as the channel through which God may become manifest.
Four.

Five.
From matter springs life. Four passes into Five. Matter diversifies into the five protrusions of a man, a budding foetus.
Five.

The path from One to Five goes through woman. She is instrumental in allowing the Word to become manifest. Through the birth of a child, a woman can partake in the Mystery of Birth and Death.

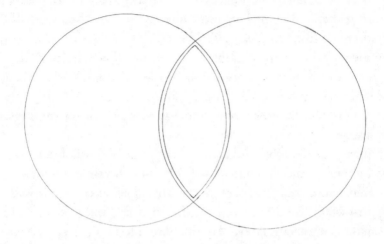

The vesica pisces is a pervasive symbol in Christianity and other religions. It is possible to look at the vesica pisces as a vagina, the opening of a birth canal. What is it that awaits us at the end of the birth canal? At the end of the dark tunnel described in near-death experiences? Birth and death, the two moments are connected like the serpent biting its tail.

Accepting your birth

Accept that your birth is as it is. The attitude 'I hope it will be as short and painless as possible' is the birth of tension, not a baby. It is a tense thought. I'll shut my eyes and tense up and *bear* the pain and then it will be over with. You cannot bear the pain. You who seek what lies at the core of the mystery of childbirth will immerse yourself, will plunge into the depths of your inner world and find a reality of a higher order than that of the material body. The experience you are offered is so much greater and of so much finer a substance that the attitude of 'bearing' it will shut you out from its true potential. Strive to accept the birthing experience for what it is. Whatever it may bring, it is what it is.

It may bring your greatest fears. Babies do die in the womb. Children die during childbirth. You have to wait until you are in your seventies before your risk of dying begins to equal that of your first week of life. Children die from cot death. Toddlers die. Teenagers die. Adults die. You too may die during childbirth. These are all possibilities, but they are not the only ones. Use your ability to see all around, from a height. Use your ability to see all the possibilities, to really see all of them, not just, as you have been conditioned, to home in on the negative possibilities.

Direct your thoughts and focus on the positive possibilities. You are not a victim of the thoughts that float through your mind. They are not even your own. If you observe yourself for sufficiently long you will begin to see this. Accept your birth for what it is and it will bring you the sweet fruit of your labour. Do not wish it to be another way. Even a disaster is a growing experience and can be immensely rich.

We plan our lives and feel perhaps more secure the more we plan. It feels like control. In fact, everything happens. We live under the law of accident. Much greater forces are at work determining our lives, but sometimes events match our expectations or plans and we are lulled into a sense that we have succeeded in realizing our plans.

Influences are all around us, from the 'collective subconscious' of all of mankind, from the stars and planets, from the geographical region and culture in which we were born and grew up, to the unquestioned behaviours resulting from imitating those around us as children.

We set out to do A and things generally start well. After a while a little change in the direction of the process occurs and we think, oh, that's so small a change it doesn't mater, it will be all right anyway. After a while, yet another little shift occurs and again we tell ourselves that we are still more or less on target. This continues, little by little, and when we eventually come to the conclusion of the process, we are convinced that this outcome is in fact what we intended at the outset. But if we examine it objectively, the outcome is actually quite different from that which we intended when we started. It doesn't feel like that because we have made the commensurate little shifts in our mind and expectations along the way, and so believe that we have had just the outcome we expected and intended.

It is an illusion that you can plan the birth of your child and your experience of it by relying on an elective caesarean. By trying to 'control' your birth in this way you will set in motion a train of events that is quite different from consciously submitting to the forces of nature.

This does not mean that you stop making efforts to attain the life, the results that you wish for. That would be madness. You have the possibility of accepting that you cannot completely control life or events. Yet you still plan and make efforts to attain the result you wish for. This is the real meaning of hope.

The I of the storm

You are the I of the storm. There is a quiet place within.

You need not be conscious in the usual sense of the word, noticing the passage of time, noticing other people's feelings and moods around you. Your sense of time alters as you progress through labour. You sink further into yourself to depths you have never seen before, to your very essence, your very nature. Let go of your 'control.' Let your body do its divine work and surrender. When the waves of contractions wash over, through you, you notice them somewhere distant, in a faraway place.

Here you will find, if you allow yourself to follow the beckoning hand of eternity, that your body allows you to become a vessel, a passage for a force so powerful that it is beyond anything we can experience in our usual state. Time disappears and you enter into the halls of eternity, the fourth dimension, that which lies beyond matter and time. Life is breathed through you and your tissues are extended to the utmost, almost dissolved, to allow this to happen.

I was giving birth to my first son, in the middle stages of labour, in an alternative birth clinic in a hospital. In my deeply meditative state I noticed the clock on the wall and a voice inside me said that I ought to pay attention to that, to check what time it was, to see how long I had been there. Was it day or night? I couldn't make sense of it; it remained merely numbers on the wall. I was blessed, outside of time, the passage of time mattered not.

Or say that the end precedes the beginning,
And the end and the beginning were always there
Before the beginning and after the end.
And all is always now. Words strain,
Crack and sometimes break, under the burden
(From 'Burnt Norton,' *Four Quartets*, T.S. Eliot)

In you, end and beginning meet. You are the closing point of the circle for the dying being, struggling to take his last breath at the end, and the being struggling to take his first breath at the beginning. In you, the circle closes, the serpent bites its tail and eternity out of time manifests through woman.

The poet recognizes this and knows that the child is still connected with a place out of place, a time out of time. The poet's intelligent emotions, which he has allowed to remain open and clean, and which he trains through his work, can see what we only vaguely recall, like a waft of scent lingering on the breeze.

Our birth is but a sleep and a forgetting:
The Soul that rises with us, our life's Star,
Hath had elsewhere its setting,
And cometh from afar:
Not in entire forgetfulness,
And not in entire nakedness,
But trailing clouds of glory do we come
From God, who is our home:
Heaven lies about us in our infancy!
Shades of the prison-house begin to close
Upon the growing Boy,
But he beholds the light, and whence it flows,
He sees it in his joy;
The Youth, who daily farther from the East
Must travel, still is Nature's Priest,
And by the vision splendid
Is on his way attended;

At length the Man perceives it die away,
And fade into the light of common day.'
(From 'Ode: Intimations of Mortality from Recollections
of Early Childhood,' William Wordsworth)

What is pain?

Pain and pleasure lie very close, right next to each other in the world
of sensation.

Pain is a signal from instinctive function that something in your
organism is not as it should be. It communicates danger and forces you
to rest or stop an activity.

In childbirth, you experience something akin to pain, but you are
not being asked to stop. You experience the overwhelming strength
and force of the transition from what was before to what will be. In
childbirth, this force, or pain, is necessary and good.

The pain of childbirth is like a vastly powerful force passing through
your body, like electricity or magnetism, yet neither. The force of
whirlwinds, storms, the power that turns planets, spins galaxies and that
opens up the universe passes through you. Any pain is the experience of
your physical body being too small, too coarse for the pressure of finer
energies passing through your flesh, through your tissues. In childbirth,
pain is being in the presence of that which is infinitely higher and more
powerful than us.

Reborn as Mother

You are not just giving birth to a child. It is absolutely necessary for you
to experience the difficulties and hardships of labour, if it is conscious
labour, in order to be born as Mother. Only that difficulty can give you
the understanding and wisdom you will need as a mother to your child.
You are being born at the same time as your child is being born, and this
applies to every subsequent child too. When a new being comes into
your circle of responsibility, becomes your kin, it shifts the balance for

everyone around you, even those only just touching upon your circle. We are not usually aware of this. The new baby changes the dynamic of your family, your relationship with your partner, with your other children, with your own mother. Once you hold the child in your arms for the first time, the world is changed forever.

Birth is the death of the woman you were, the end of all that was before and the beginning of a new life in the world. You, being given the unique privilege of existing in this world as Mother, need to be born and reborn in ever increasing degrees of strength and wisdom, to act as the pivot around which your family orbits. Can you hold your children as gently and firmly as the sun holds its planets? Can you let them be themselves fully yet know just where to draw in the reins? Can you let them be the growing branch of the universe, the one harbouring all the potential?

You need to undergo this trial by fire in order to become the person you need to be for the next stage of your life: Mother, or Mother of two, or Mother of three. Nature has in its great design allowed for each mother to experience just what is necessary for her to become the mother she needs to be. You are the transforming enzyme of your family. This is a great honour and a responsibility. Be the queen you are, hold your head high, for you are the still hub of the spinning wheel of family life.

Perhaps you have noticed that women, after they have become mothers, look quite different. They can look serene, softer, more womanly, more compassionate. More tired, yes, and also more wise. A new depth of understanding, of being, has been born. A new Self has emerged.

7. Practical Considerations During Birth

The practical considerations relating to giving birth are of paramount importance. They can make the difference between a traumatic birth and a smooth one, between a safe birth and a life-threatening scenario. Don't underestimate the importance of the little things in life. The sum total of all the little things we do is our overall experience, what happens to us. So we can have an influence on what happens to us by taking responsibility for the little practicalities.

Food

The first thing is: be prepared. Make sure that, *as soon as labour begins*, the birthing mother eats a bowl of pasta or porridge. This will give you the slow-release energy that you will need during labour. It's good to eat as early as possible as you may feel sick later and may not be able to eat at all.

The feeding of the birthing mother is very important, perhaps the most important contribution your partner can make to a good birth. Offer her frequent small doses of fruit sugars, such as glucose tablets, together with sips of water. Water can be offered every five minutes, between contractions; fruit sugars every twenty minutes or so. This consistent sustenance will help to prevent exhaustion and is a major contributor to a safe birth. It has been shown that women who are well-hydrated have faster, smoother labours than those who are not.

If you push yourself to keep going through the contractions and the intense muscular work your womb has to go through without replenishing your resources, you will soon be exhausted and lose your judgment. Labour may then slow down and the child may become distressed. This can manifest itself in a reduced heartbeat, which could then trigger a chain of events characterized by panic, fear and interference in the birthing process.

The importance of your birthing partner

Your partner needs to be ready to respond to any request the mother might make: for a blanket, for the room temperature to be adjusted, for some cold water in the birthing pool, for a sweet, nourishing drink (like rosehip syrup), for music to be turned off. Childbirth is extremely hard work and may make you feel much hotter than those around you. These things may seem small and insignificant, but they are not; they are the little boosts and nudges that keep the process going in the right direction.

Be prepared that any offer of help may be robustly rejected: 'NO!!! **** OFF! I DIDN'T ****ING WANT *THAT*!' is par for the course and your partner must not allow themself to be put off. Their job is to remain balanced, calm and strong and to act as a point of security and nourishment for the mother. During birth, they are the Moon to the woman's Earth, revolving around her and acting as a counterweight, maintaining balance and equilibrium. Let it be water off a hero's back.

Movement

Feel free to move around freely if it feels right, as moving has been demonstrated to help the birth progress quickly and smoothly. Sway and rock and allow yourself to move with the rhythm of your birth.

Breathing

Make noise, go with your breath and with your urge to make noise. Do not hold back. Low like a cow, bellow, grunt and moan if you want. The noises you make during childbirth seem to come from an ancient place deep within you; they do not seem to be made with your ordinary voice. Expel your breath fully. A Buddhist monk has helpfully questioned why we westerners are so frightened of exhaling. If you give a little attention to your breathing, without changing it, you will see that you spend a large part of your life not breathing as deeply as you would if you were fully relaxed. What is this tension that keeps us from living our lives fully — restricts us and inhibits our instinctive and emotional functions? It is a question worth pondering.

The physiology of tension and fear lowers our threshold for pain. If your muscles are tense and taut they are more likely to tear or suffer injury. If you are knotted up inside you have no resources left for dealing with heightened sensation or pain. Tension exacerbates pain and discomfort, and if we are not prepared, pain in turn exacerbates tension and a vicious cycle may take form. During birth, let it be your role to not hold back; don't try and control your breath or your expression. Let the birthing force flow through you freely. Go with it.

It can be helpful to research breathing techniques. The following practice is known to be helpful to some women: As soon as a contraction begins to sweep through you, inhale deeply and slowly through your nose and then let the air flow out gently through pursed lips, as if you were blowing out a candle. Try to continue this for the full length of the contraction. This is helpful because it ensures that you breathe deeply and slowly during contractions. It also helps you to go with the force sweeping through your body and the ensuing discomfort.

If you decide to do this, make sure that you practise it beforehand. It is worth spending some time preparing and trying it out together with your partner. Practice allows a series of movements, small or big, to pass from your intellect, which is slow, to your responsive and capable moving function. By the time birth comes, you will not need to apply your intellect to remember what you were supposed to do. This can be more difficult than you think! Do not underestimate the slowness of the intellect in a crisis, and use your wonderful instinctive-moving function to do the job for you.

Anyone who has learned to ride a bike or play the piano, or even to read can understand this. For example, you do not cycle with your intellect. Your intellect instructs the moving function to begin with, but once your moving function has got it, it takes over and is much better at cycling than your intellect. Try to cycle whilst being intellectually aware of every movement: pedalling, steering, balancing. Then just let your moving function do it!

It is important to breathe deeply throughout your contractions. Breathing deeply brings nourishment and oxygen into your baby's body, as well as releasing carbon dioxide and reducing stress. It is helpful, if not essential, to both you and your baby during childbirth. Taking slow, deep breaths will help to make your birth both safer and less painful.

It's easy to fall into a pattern of short, gasping breaths if you have not prepared your breathing. When we hurt ourselves we tend to gasp and hold our breath while the pain subsides. This may work when the injury is minor, like a burn or a pin-prick, and in any case it is an unconscious reflex. However, it is most unhelpful during birth, when we need to take deep, slow breaths despite experiencing pain and discomfort. The unconscious reflex of gasping for breath can be made to serve a purpose if we use it to observe ourselves; start by trying to become aware of when you react like this.

The environment of birth

Your prepared birthing space, which might be a darkened room, can help you to focus, to go within and to let labour flow through you. So seek out a darkened, quiet ambience when you are ready. Allow yourself to begin to sink into the deep peace that lies within.

When under the immense pressure of childbirth, every unfamiliar thing, sight, sound and smell is a burden on your system and drains vital resources away from birthing. If you give birth in a familiar environment you will have a significant advantage. You need not expend an ounce of energy on orientating yourself in a building or a room, finding where a noise is coming from or what that smell is. You will be secure, you can know what to expect from creaking doors, slippery carpets and dodgy drains. They are your dodgy drains, you are familiar with them, they are your reference point and are not a cause of stress.

This kind of stress may seem negligible, but as anyone who has attended a birth can attest, it is not so. Just changing the music or switching the lights on or off can elicit an outburst of expletives from the birthing mother.

You will know, subconsciously or consciously, where the compass points are in each room, where the sun comes in and how it moves across your familiar objects. You will know where the escape routes are, where the front door is, if there is a path at the back of the house. All this is part of your subconscious awareness of your environment and it contributes to making you feel safe, and thereby relaxed, at home.

To try to reproduce a home environment in a hospital by furnishing a room with homely objects, then expect women to reap the full benefits of home birth, as is done in some hospitals, appears naïve. It is reminiscent of the disconcerting horror of the 'home-like' environment reproduced in the alien zoo in Stanley Kubrick's *2001 — A Space Odyssey.*

The hospital environment presents other challenges too. The midwives' shift changes are horrendously stressful. Just when you feel that you may be able to cope with this immensely difficult and entirely new and shocking experience, the person who was your anchor in the storm clocks off. It can be traumatic.

Labour can slow down significantly as a result of a shift change. The midwife who comes to work the next shift may not be right for you, even if the first one was. You may never have set eyes on either of them before. A number of hours pass and you gradually grow accustomed to this person, you begin to hammer out a working relationship, and then she leaves too. This is so stressful as to be almost inhuman, and is certainly counterproductive from a medical perspective. There must be a better way, even in hospitals. During a home birth, the midwife stays with you until the child is born.

Hospital personnel are trained to focus on medical procedures, not on emotional obstacles that can be removed, or psychological fears that can be overcome, or the intellectual formulation of a process. The focus lies on jargon, technology and procedure. Mechanical man has produced a mechanical behemoth that dispenses mechanical treatment. We have the potential to be more than machines, but first we have to acknowledge that in some ways that is what we are.

The Midwife

This is a calling. It is a calling to assist a mother as she reaches down into the depths of herself and into the mysteries of the universe, to guide her, to help her past obstacles, physical and psychological, to coax, encourage and reassure her, and to remain a point of detachment and calm.

The midwife allows the mother to have the birth that she wants, is sensitive and assists each mother differently according to her needs. The midwife has extensive anatomical, medical and pharmaceutical knowledge. She knows all the points of contact with doctors, hospitals and emergency services. She is aware of all the practical needs of the birth, such as food, clean cloths, noise, light etc. At the same time she is tuned into where the mother is, physiologically and psychologically.

She may remain entirely in the background and say virtually nothing and yet be of the utmost assistance to a birthing mother. She may tell you to shout all the profanities you know at the top of your voice as you push, to release your full power and remove any last inhibitions. She is fully present. She understands the stages of labour and has seen many different births progress and go through their unique and universal rhythms again and again.

A midwife is both priestess and doctor, and closer to the healing profession than many a highly-qualified medical specialist. She is also a woman. She has a womb. She has had periods. She has a clitoris, labia and breasts. There is an instinctive understanding that comes from that. She is not just a coach. She will stay with you from when you call her until the placenta is delivered.

Search until you find such a midwife. There are many but they are not commonplace. In preparation for the birth of my second child in Sweden, I did my own research and eventually found a midwife who I connected with and who was willing to work with me privately. Taking responsibility for your birthing experience requires effort; not just taking no for an answer, and not just accepting what we are told is 'best' for us.

The surprise

The moment of birth, when you hold your child in your arms for the first time, can, oddly, be one of great surprise. You would have thought it hardly surprising that a baby lies at the end of pregnancy and labour, but that really is the feeling that can emerge when your child is born. 'Oh my God, a baby. I'm not sure I was really expecting that. I'm in a bit of a kerfuffle now. Is this where I am now?' Perhaps the father can see more clearly, from outside: 'He, my child, has come.'

Although you have thought so much and prepared so much and dreamed so much about this birth, the real moment is not what you had expected or imagined, because it is real. The baby is not this sweet thing, a figment of your imagination, but a real and complete person, and oddly, he is more complete than yourself. We recognize this at some deep level, when we gaze into his eyes and see that he knows all the mysteries and precisely why he has come. Yet *you* have got to take care of and be responsible for *him*. This is deeply surprising. It is unsettling and awakening.

This new being entering the world has changed it forever and you can feel the weight, the significance of this for a few moments after birth. Then life takes over again and you become preoccupied with caring for your child, just as you should.

8. Home Birth

Hospitals look at birth, implicitly, as a process where things may go wrong and where the hospital can then offer help. This is simply a result of the way we live today and all the unspoken assumptions that underpin it. There is obviously no deliberate, evil manipulation of women. However, this approach means that in a hospital environment, the doctors, nurses and midwives who work there are constantly on the lookout for problems to be rectified. This will attract 'problems,' draw attention to 'problems' and, as everyone is motivated by their understanding of what is good, hospital procedures will be initiated at the earliest opportunity. A woman in labour is viewed as a patient, on a par with other patients whose bodies are not functioning as they should.

More appropriate than focusing on possible illness and injury, is an underlying attitude of devotion, one of honouring woman and the mysteries that she embodies during birth. This does not mean that medical expertise is not necessary, or that all drugs or surgical procedures should be avoided at any cost. This is a very important point; it is not one or the other, it is one *and* the other.

The real world cannot be reached in the way that we have become accustomed to think. Not through yes or no, down or up, right or wrong. It is easy and tempting to count no further than to two. It is more demanding and also more becoming as a human being to strive to synthesize. Count all the way to three and you will learn to recognize how easy it is to follow the path of least resistance. Dead fish float downstream with ease. The living swim upstream with effort, working against the current, against the friction of the moving water and towards life: towards reproduction, towards germinating their seed, towards fulfilling their potential.

If there are complications during a hospital birth the response you are likely to get from those around you is that you were really lucky to have given birth in hospital when things went wrong. If you research this, however, you will find that things have often gone wrong as a result of hospital intervention. A planned home birth is very safe, arguably safer than a hospital birth.

If you choose to have a home birth you will probably want to establish the position of the foetus in the weeks before birth. If it turns out to be feet or bottom first, you might want to try to turn the baby around. Speak to your midwife and make sure that everything feels right ahead of the birth. Assume responsibility for your own birth.

The risks of home birth

If you tell people that you are having a home birth the reaction is often, 'What if something goes wrong?' What is implicit in this question? Is it that avoiding difficulties *at any cost* is the unquestionable desired goal? Karma yoga is the practice of refraining from trying to avoid difficulties. It is to choose not to follow the path of least resistance. Karma yoga is the practice of transforming the tableaux presented to you in life, *your* experiences, into something profitable for you, for the growth of your soul and for those around you. To do this, we need to begin to know ourselves, to become familiar with our habitual attempts at avoiding difficulty. The illusion of life (Maya) is that we can avoid difficulty. The truth is that we will encounter it whether we try to avoid it or not. Our true potential lies in this possibility of actively entering into difficulty. This represents our potential to transform human suffering into something finer, into something higher. To climb the ladder that leads all the way up to Heaven.

Although some women do give birth alone, and this can undoubtedly be a tremendously empowering experience, it is common sense to rely on a good midwife, someone who is experienced and able to deal with emergencies and complications. Find out exactly what equipment she will have with her. It will probably not be very much, but it will still be everything you could possibly need for a normal birth and most complications. As you are taking responsibility for your own birth, rather than handing yourself over to the 'experts,' you will probably want to know what this equipment is.

Do your own research regarding the risks of hospital births and home births. Study the statistics, find out about different methods, consider the possible scenarios. You need to find out for yourself.

Sheila Kitzinger's excellent book *Homebirth* is a classic. It tells you just about everything you need to know about home birth. She concludes that, 'The perinatal mortality rate for planned home births is very low — 3–4 per thousand compared with 9–10 births as a whole.'

The vast majority of all learning disabilities in babies already exist before labour sets in. It is worth addressing the possibility that you give birth to a very ill baby that will die within hours or days. If this is the case, how would you wish this to unfold? Where, in what atmosphere? In what surroundings? Think about it and consider the possibility of your baby dying hooked up to equipment and with lots of unknown people milling about, with stress and fear in the air. Ponder it carefully and take responsibility.

Remember that she wanted to come. She chose to come even though she knew what would happen. It was worthwhile, for precisely what reason we cannot know, but she came, was born, came into being and went again.

> *And all shall be well, and*
> *All manner of thing shall be well*
> (From 'Little Gidding,' *Four Quartets*, T.S. Eliot)

In intensive care units in hospitals there are many babies that should perhaps be allowed to go whence they have come in peace, but are being kept artificially alive, at the cost of considerable suffering in the child, and only *because it is possible* to sustain life by artificial means. Insight and maturity are not easily come by, and the great mechanical colossus that is healthcare in our civilization does not always show these attributes. Include such possible outcomes in your careful consideration of how you wish to give birth.

Your own preparation will avoid most complications. Relaxation, assurance and acceptance are the keys to a good birth.

Your partner and the midwife are the ideal minimum number of attendants. In an emergency, two people may be needed. Use your imagination, but intelligently and actively, so that it does not run away with more possible negative scenarios than common sense suggests. Assess these possible scenarios that your controlled imagination presents, assess them dispassionately. You will probably come to the conclusion that a minimum of two people will need to be present at your birth.

When you are an experienced birther, when you know your body in childbirth well, when it is your third or fourth baby that is coming, then, perhaps, you will feel differently. I gave birth to my third child with only my husband there for support. The birth was so smooth that I didn't call the midwife until about an hour before my baby was actually born. By the time the midwife had arrived, all I had to do was to give one final push. The midwife didn't have time to examine me or listen to the baby's heartbeat; all she needed to do was to confirm that this was the birth of a happy, healthy boy at home.

Obviously you will need to be able to get to hospital in a dire emergency; this is your right and one of the real advantages of living in the industrialized west. It is easy to be romantic about a simple life but, mechanistic as it may be, the west has reached many valuable understandings and implemented them effectively, only without understanding the whole.

Maintain a good level of cleanliness in your home before the birth. If, prior to the birth, you give the rooms you will be using a good clean and prepare clean towels and have access to hot water, this will be more than adequate. This will probably come naturally to you as your instinctive function knows the importance of this. You are likely to want to keep things fastidiously clean and tidy and may feel an overwhelming urge to sort out all your old cupboards and boxes before the birth. This is an excellent opportunity to observe the work of your instinctive function and how it communicates with your intellectual function.

Birth can be messy, so you may want to cover your carpets and furniture with sheets or plastic in preparation.

The primary risk of home birth is probably that of self-reproach if something 'goes wrong.' Take responsibility. Paradoxically, this means to let go of the illusion that you can control life.

Water birth

It can be extremely helpful, relaxing and soothing to get into warm water when labour has progressed to a more difficult stage. Hundreds of thousands of women around the world have given birth in water and benefited from its calming and pain-relieving effect. It is possible to receive your child with your own hands in a birthing pool at home. Some women find that water slows the labour down, and it's not right for everyone. Explore, research and choose according to your own needs and wishes.

In some countries water birth is strongly discouraged and it may not even be possible to get hold of a birthing pool. This reflects the view of some parts of the medical establishment that water birth is dangerous. It certainly does not appear natural for a land-living animal to give birth in water. Nevertheless the promise of getting into the water when labour is getting difficult to manage can help you tremendously.

Listen to yourself and think for yourself. Do what you feel is right for you.

If you are planning a home water birth you need to take into account the purity of the water that you will be using. You may be lucky and have a large water storage tank or combi-boiler that will provide enough warm water to fill the birthing pool. If not, you need to find another way of ensuring that you always have enough warm, clean water to fill the pool when it is required.

In my case, the hot water tank only provided sufficient hot water to fill a quarter of the birthing pool, so my husband and I rented cement heaters from a building supply firm, which we cleaned and disinfected.

My husband affixed these heating elements to a wooden frame over the birthing pool to keep the water at a constant temperature of 37°C (98.5°F). The birthing pool was cleaned and disinfected before filling it with water. The water was changed every 24 hours. We added sea salt to the clean water to act as a natural disinfectant. Use your common sense — it is a greatly underrated faculty.

9. Hospital Birth

The risks of hospital birth

If you give birth in hospital, there are three primary risks:

1. Your labour may not proceed naturally or normally because of the stress caused by the unfamiliar environment, by people coming and going and by routine tests being made.

   Your labour might start, then stop, then start again, then stop, which is exhausting for you and your baby. This may then trigger hospital procedures, such as: if a woman has not dilated fully within twelve hours the recommended course of action is to induce birth. The aim is to make your labour conform to a norm. The stress may be further exacerbated by the unfamiliar surroundings, the reactions of people who don't know you and who may express negativity or exhibit an unsupportive attitude, interference from equipment and professionals as well as bright lights and noise.

2. The risk of infection. A normally clean home will contain much fewer bacteria than a hospital.

   The fact is that MRSA and other abnormally strong bacterial life tend to develop in a hospital environment, not in the home.

3. Serious complications may arise as a result of hospital intervention
   such as induction, pharmaceutical pain relief or mechanical
   intervention like caesarean section or the use of forceps.

As soon as you start a process of medical interference, one thing
triggers another and you will soon have abandoned the chain of natural
birthing events.

Induction

Birth can be induced by introducing artificial oxytocin (pitocin) into
the woman's bloodstream, applying prostaglandin gel to the cervix or
by rupturing the foetal sack so that the amniotic fluid begins to escape
('breaking your waters'). This means that your baby may be forced to
enter the world before he is ready for life.

'Active management' is a term used by some medical professionals to
describe procedures that ensure that a birth conforms to certain norms.
Such norms might be that a mother is 'permitted' a maximum of twelve
hours in labour, a minimum of one centimetre dilation of the cervix
per hour or a maximum of one hour of pushing before birth is induced.
Surveys have established that routine induction increases the job
satisfaction of obstetricians and makes it easier to run maternity wards.

Of course there are medically justified exceptions, such as in pre-
eclampsia, when a woman's blood pressure becomes dangerously high
and the placenta may be unable to support the baby's life. Then it may
be a good idea to induce the birth.

Because the method of introducing oxytocin into the bloodstream
by a drip is so crude compared to the delicate work and considered
response of the endocrinal glands inside the body, labour may be much
more intense and fast than it would otherwise have been, like running
a moped on rocket fuel. This implies considerably more pain for the
woman giving birth.

The woman may become so disturbed, so out of synch with her
natural rhythm of labour, that she ends up demanding medical pain

relief where she would otherwise not have done so. This will be readily given, of course, as it justifies the importance of providing it and increases job satisfaction: 'I can do something to help this poor suffering woman.'

Once an epidural has been given, the woman may need a catheter inserted into her bladder as she may not be able to feel the need to urinate. This increases the risk of infection. She is now in a position where she can no longer walk. This is likely to slow down labour further as moving about has been shown to assist labour. The quantity of artificial oxytocin then has to be increased further and the vicious circle continues.

It is also worth considering that an intravenous drip may introduce excess fluid into the woman's body that alters her metabolic balance. In extreme cases, this has been known to result in the woman experiencing convulsions.

Induction can also force the uterus to overdo its work, with unnaturally strong and long contractions, restricting the baby's blood flow. Normal contractions gently squeeze the baby downwards. Induced contractions are more akin to a clamping machine. There is a risk that the uterus goes into spasm, which can then affect the baby's heartbeat.

For you, personally, the experience is that you are chained to equipment, with a needle in your arm, a catheter in your bladder, possibly a monitoring electrode coming out of your vagina and a plastic tube for topping up the epidural coming out of your back. Is this the way to experience the most miraculous event of womanhood? You are reduced to being a victim, helpless, monitored, unable to trust your own feelings and sensations about what is going on in your body. Machines are consulted before you. You are separated from your child before she is even born.

The baby's heartbeat may be so closely monitored that it adds to the mother's stress rather than relieving it. Every beat is registered, watched anxiously on a flashing and beeping machine. Use your imagination to really envisage this situation. Use your intellect to deduce the possible consequences. This is likely to make the mother tense and to slow down the natural progression further. If the heart rate changes significantly, further medical intervention will take place regardless of what the mother's intuition tells her. The machine will almost certainly be deemed to know better.

Childbirth is initiated by the baby himself, when he is ready. Failing to trust him may make for a perilous start to his life here on earth. Again, there will naturally be instances where induction is the best, or even only, course of action, but these are rare exceptions. If you listen to your common sense, you will see that the overwhelming majority of births do not need to be induced.

If it is necessary for you to be induced, then so be it. You are prepared and you know what you are doing. No one is unintentionally manipulating you to give birth in a way that you do not want. You go into it with your eyes open and it is good.

Your birth is your birth, and whatever it brings is exactly right for you and your child; it is what is needed for your development at this time. When you're driving along in your car, you don't constantly check the rear-view mirror to keep track of what your earlier manoeuvres have resulted in. No, you look forwards, towards what is coming, and cast a glance in the rear-view mirror now and then to see that nothing unexpected is going to catch you unawares from behind. It is possible for this to apply to your life experiences: keep your eyes on the road ahead and don't dwell on what has been. This book is about how you can prepare for the birth that you want, and if reality does not match your expectations, then reality is right. That is precisely what should have been. It is what it is.

Risks of pharmaceutical pain relief

Pharmaceutical pain relief is offered in hospitals during labour and includes opiates such as pethidine, epidurals and nitrous oxide (gas and air).

Inhaled nitrous oxide is usually offered in the first instance. It can cause light-headedness and nausea, and should ideally not be used throughout labour.

Pethidine is often administered if nitrous oxide gas does not relieve the pain. Studies have shown that it is often unsatisfactory as a means of pain relief, and common side effects include vomiting and dizziness, which significantly impair the mother's birthing experience. Mother and child become sleepy, affecting the crucial first moments of sustained eye contact and bonding.

Pethidine crosses the placenta to reach the foetus, and can cause respiratory depression, impair the baby's ability to move and compromise breastfeeding. Because some of the baby's internal functioning is not yet fully developed, the drug has a stronger effect on the baby. Before birth, the mother's liver processes the drug, but once the baby is born the baby's immature liver has to take over. For more than a month after birth, babies with high pethidine exposure are more likely to cry when handled, and it reduces the infant's ability to quiet himself once aroused.

Diamorphine is a more powerful narcotic that is also sometimes offered during labour.

Epidural analgesia is given by injection into the spine and has been shown to be effective in relieving labour pains. Epidural analgesia frequently prolongs labour and leads to further intervention such as forceps delivery, because the mother loses sensation and her ability to push is compromised.

Epidural analgesia crosses the placenta and enters the foetus, and epidural babies are far more likely to be investigated and admitted for neonatal care.

Epidurals tend to raise the birthing mother's temperature, leading doctors to suspect that their babies have an infection at birth. Epidural babies are nearly five times as likely to be evaluated for sepsis, which can involve lumbar punctures as well as administering antibiotics. The mother and baby will then be separated in those first crucial moments.

Forceps

Forceps are a tong-like instrument used in hospitals for grasping the baby's head during labour. A suction cup can also be used. To attach the instrument to the baby's head an incision (episiotomy) is made through the back wall of the vagina into the perineum (the area between the vagina and the rectum).

The incision implies a risk of the wound becoming infected and increased risk of urinary tract infection. The incision can also lead to severe tearing in the vaginal wall, which can leave the mother faecally incontinent. Forceps deliveries are also associated with a greater risk of losing a lot of blood and needing a blood transfusion.

Risks to the baby associated with forceps delivery include bruising the baby's face, damage to the baby's facial nerves, skull or collarbone fractures, spinal cord injury and cerebral palsy. Babies born by forceps have sometimes been reported to be demanding and difficult to comfort. Cranial osteopaths claim that a lot of their work is done with babies whose skull bones appear to have become misaligned as a result of forceps birth.

The suction cup implies an increased risk of bleeding in the brain.

Episiotomies

An episiotomy is where an incision is made to enlarge the opening of the vagina. This may be imposed on a woman giving birth in hospital if her tissues are considered not to have stretched sufficiently, itself a possible result of all the unnatural conditions imposed on the woman's body. Episiotomies are painful and can lead to blood loss and resulting fatigue in a woman already under extreme stress.

Episiotomies are sometimes performed without anaesthesia or without waiting for the anaesthetic to work properly, as a result of the panicked situation caused by interference. Of course, infection is also a risk. It is worthwhile considering that there is a higher risk of a further tear in the anus and rectum after an episiotomy compared to when a tear occurs naturally. The pain after a tear caused naturally is significantly less than that following an episiotomy.

I tore during the births of my first and second child, a few centimetres each time, and did not experience any significant pain when it happened, in fact I didn't notice it. Afterwards, I was sore when I went to the toilet for four or five days and then it quickly got better. The tears were left to heal naturally, I had no stitches, and when my third child came along I didn't tear at all.

Because the wound caused by an episiotomy will always be stitched, it is possible that the stitching may be done too tightly, without leaving enough room for swelling. In very sensitive tissues, such as those around the vagina, swelling tends to be more pronounced than in other tissues. More women experience pain when making love after an episiotomy than those with a natural tear.

Some women may experience a perforation of the wall separating the vagina from the rectum and may pass faeces through the vaginal opening and so require further surgery during the first six months. This is a crucial period when you are getting to know your baby and yourself as a mother. Such an experience may contribute to post-natal depression and may even lead to the woman feeling that she has been violated.

Most surveys show an increased risk of more serious tears in women who undergo episiotomies. Studies have also shown that the position you adopt during birth significantly influences the risk of tearing, although there is no ideal position for all women. You will need to listen to your body, your instincts and intuition to find the situation that works best for you.

Episiotomies are at best necessary in very rare and life-threatening circumstances, and at worst the cruel maiming of an otherwise healthy woman, causing unnecessary suffering and complicating the present and future births.

There are considerable risks associated with induction, pharmaceutical pain relief and mechanical interference and you should carefully consider these possible outcomes before you decide where and how you give birth.

Electronic foetal monitoring

In electronic foetal monitoring two electronic sensors are placed on the top of your stomach, and are held in place with elastic belts. They use ultrasound to monitor your contractions and your baby's heartbeat.

In high-risk cases, a small clip called a foetal scalp electrode may be placed on your baby's head instead to monitor his heartbeat. If the mother's waters have not yet broken, in order to attach an electrode to a baby's skull, it's necessary to rupture the membranes of the amniotic sack, allowing amniotic fluid to seep out. This compromises the sterile environment in the amniotic sac and reduces the cushioning effect of the amniotic fluid on the baby, which can restrict blood flow from the placenta to the baby.

The attention is then focused on a machine displaying data. The midwife or doctor may come in, look at the machine and say that everything is fine. Your partner may be asked to keep an eye on the machine while they are out of the room. How is this going to make the woman feel? Her impression of the birth, her sensations and intuitions are not even considered.

Caesarean section

Caesarean delivery implies an increased risk of death compared to natural childbirth. Having a caesarean implies a substantially increased risk of infection, will necessitate a longer hospital stay and is more likely to result in you needing a blood transfusion. These are the facts.

Children who have been born naturally, through the vagina, and have received some traces of bacteria from the mother's faeces, are less likely to develop allergies later in life than those born by caesarean section.

There is an argument that it is a woman's right to choose freely what kind of birth she wants, be it caesarean or natural. However, being able to do what you want is not necessarily the same as being free.

One of the difficulties we face as a result of the way we live today is that we are continuously trying to substitute outer freedom for inner freedom. Inner freedom is not dependent on your circumstances. Outer freedom, the pursuit of ever more detailed choice, is a chimera. You never get there. There is always something more to be had, to be bought or to be aspired to. These days there is no limit to our choices, so we are hypnotized further into the delusion that we are free to choose what our life will be like. We never actually begin to live, because we are always trying to improve our lot. This is a major cause of the increase in depression and burn-out in our time.

Have you ever wondered how you became the person you are? The person that wants this and does not want that; likes him but does not like her: that person is largely the result of imitation. Unconsciously, you imitate your parents and others. Observe a child and see how readily he seeks out role models, copying gesture, posture and intonation. The child is so open, vulnerable, trusting, so very eager to learn from us. Education continues the process of substituting the accumulation of knowledge for acting in accordance with conscience.

Education fills us with answers, and sometimes puts a stop to our questioning. That within us which seeks the truth about our origins begins to atrophy. Ready-made answers are given in school and continue to be given all the way to university. 'In Ancient Greece, people believed xxx. Now, of course, we *know* that it is yyy.' Learn the facts. Be knowledgeable about what others have said or thought. The child, being innocent and trusting, does his best to live up to the expectations of those around him.

That in you, or in anyone, that wants an elective caesarean is not you. It has been pasted onto you over many years. We are encouraged to cater to our every whim by shopping and spending and buying and consuming, satisfying the needs of the lowest part of us. Media, TV, newspapers, magazines, catalogues tell us this, ceaselessly. We are upside down. The lowest part is king and has the full run of our father's house. The highest part is pushed down into the basement, in the dark, separated from the rest of us: the subconscious.

However, it does not mean that that is who we are. If you had been subjected to none of this, who would you be? Can you begin to see that the desire to have an elective caesarean to shield yourself from discomfort may not be your own idea? And if it is not your own idea, are you free?

You have something in you that is infinitely precious and valuable, only it is covered in caked-on dirt. You carry around with you the residue of generations. Can you sometimes see your mother in yourself? She is not you. You have copied. She has copied.

Your child, when he comes, recognizes your true Self. He has not yet begun to copy, to imitate, to become covered in habits, behaviours and the residue of generations. What is truly yours is beyond words, beyond time. You can see that recognition in your newborn child's eyes.

Treatment of newborns in hospitals

In hospital, a patient or a baby is viewed as someone with the potential for being treated. Because people who work in hospitals are motivated by a wish to help others, they are likely to want to help as soon as they possibly can. Their idea of helping a patient or a baby will be to put their expertise and equipment to its best use in the individual case.

So the motivation of the person providing medical examinations or using equipment is not malicious, it is based on that person's understanding of love or doing good. Keeping this in mind will help you to refrain from resenting individuals, and instead thinking independently and making your own decisions, not based on anger or resentment but on critical thinking, emotional understanding and physical intuition.

In hospitals, it is practice to clamp the umbilical cord within thirty seconds of birth in order to reduce the risk of mothers bleeding to death. Cutting the cord so soon after birth halts the baby's oxygen supply through the mother's blood before independent breathing has become securely established. Early cord clamping has been linked to brain haemorrhaging, iron deficiencies and mental impairment.

Many hospitals suction newborn babies to remove mucus from their nose and throat. If this is done as a routine measure, rather than a necessary procedure to save the baby's life, it should be questioned. This is a very tender and fragile moment, when the baby has just drawn its first breath or is about to and has just come into the world. This kind of brutal, mechanical action should only be used as a last resort. In some cases, it has been known to cause an irregular heartbeat in the baby. Bacteria can also be introduced into the baby's delicate breathing passages.

Other medical intervention performed on babies includes pumping their stomachs as soon as they are born. This can slow the heart rate and interfere with the baby's pattern of sucking and swallowing. Not a good start for breastfeeding.

In some hospitals, babies are still separated from their mothers at birth. Even if the baby can stay with you just after it has been born, it will often be removed and taken to a brightly-lit room to be weighed and measured after a while. At home you can do this yourself with the help of the midwife, using cloths that smell of you to wrap the baby in while it is being weighed, right there, with you.

In hospital, staff may be trained to observe you to see that you are bonding properly with your child. This kind of police state mindset can only add to the stress of the new mother and hinder a process that will take the time it takes.

Furthermore, if hospital routines dictate that a baby should be given an examination one hour after birth, say, staff will have to follow this rule rather than use their own judgment. To make the right decision about the timing of any examination, it is necessary to look at the whole picture. It is necessary to look with empathy and conscience at the mother and child, who may just have started bonding, or just started breastfeeding, or some other emotional or intangible factor which might override the need for a medical examination just then.

If you are giving birth at home, try to arrange for a doctor to visit you at home within 24 hours of the birth for a full check-up.

Another consideration

It is easy to become all 'anti' and reject *everything* that modern science and healthcare has to offer — to pretend that you can return to some imaginary Earth Mother myth where you give birth squatting on an earthen floor in the flicker of candlelight while shamans chant around you. It is too easy. This, too, is floating down the stream with the dead fish; you're just floating with another kind of fish.

When we strive to synthesize, we begin to count to three. This requires effort and intelligent use of our creative and intellectual powers. 'Alternative' can sometimes be little more than a fancy name for a reaction, and a reaction counts only to two: good and bad. Being responsible means counting to three.

Our attitudes to childbirth, if we address them and examine them dispassionately, will reveal our attitudes to many other things. They have the potential to show us what we are.

10. Breastfeeding and Lying-in

Transitional period/lying-in

We have seen that rites of passage are rituals created by conscious people to help make the existence of the great mass of humanity a little more bearable. Someone, a real person, who came to see what woman and child needed by working on themselves, by perfecting themselves, established the custom of lying-in.

Such rites of passage are a tradition, a cultural habit which members of society can follow to their benefit regardless of whether they are actually conscious of its benefits or not. Other rites of passage established by conscious people include marriage, baptism, funerals, coming-of-age rituals and periods of mourning.

However, many of these carefully constructed rites are being destroyed in the name of progress. Lying-in is one of them. There are no obvious signs on a house or in the dress of a woman or her family that she is in the lying-in period. We are in fact encouraged to get back to 'normal' as soon as possible: to lose weight, to get into the routine of caring for the baby, to get into the swing of things, even to go back to work as soon as possible.

Establishing a routine for your baby without first having spent ample time observing and getting to know the individual now in your care, and who has voluntarily placed her fully formed self entirely at your mercy, is unfeeling and mechanical. The underlying assumption is that there is no individuality in your child and that routines can be the same for everyone.

Any new mother who has gazed into the eyes of her newborn, while being fully present herself and not shackled by fear or worry, knows that her child is unique. She is a fully formed being living in a tiny and as yet incompetent body who sees the imperfections of her mother, yet lovingly allows herself to be placed in her care. These eyes speak of intelligence beyond what any of us possess, of love without conditions, of positive emotion: an emotion that cannot turn negative regardless of what happens. This needs to be acknowledged, recognized and a mutual relationship established between the two.

The emotional function of your child needs to be developed and maintained and you, the mother, are uniquely positioned to experience this privilege. Emotion, which is abstract, comes into the world through physical bodies. Your baby's emotional function needs to be built, with your help, so that conscious love may come into the realm of matter. This is only possible through a human being with fully-formed instinctive, emotional and intellectual functions. Building and maintaining emotional function take time. To assess, as is done in hospitals, whether a mother is bonding with her baby a few hours or even minutes after birth, is absurd. Why the rush?

Traditionally, a new mother is given a period of forty days to recover from the birth and bond with her new baby. Others, mainly experienced older women, take care of her, providing her with nourishing food to build her strength and to prevent milk production from being too much of a strain. The mother needs to be nurtured herself so that she can in turn nurture her child. These more experienced women help and advise the new mother on breastfeeding and caring for her child. They are around to help her with the practicalities of life, cooking and cleaning, until she is strong enough, has bonded with her baby and is ready to establish routines that suit the unique individuals in that family.

These forty days are normal for childbirth. It is abnormal when a woman is expected to be back at work after two weeks, as can be the case in the US, or where a woman is expected to be slim within weeks of giving birth. An obsession with losing weight quickly is quite selfish. Where are the reserves from which the mother can produce ample breast milk? Perhaps some women express the fear that they are not producing enough milk because they are pushed into losing weight by unspoken expectations. The fatty tissues that are intended by nature in her wisdom to act as reserves and a source of nutrition are being depleted before time.

With the birth of a child the entire family is transformed, the dynamic of relationships shifts. There is another person in the world; before there were perhaps only two of you. Now there is a new unit, a new whole, comprising three parts, with a different balance of interrelationships, of behavioural patterns and dynamics. This applies to the birth of each new child, not just the first. This is no small thing and the transformation takes time. This is a transitional phase, a period of transformation, from being a married couple to becoming a family, or from being a family of three to a family of four. Every birth changes the dynamic of life for family members and needs to be acknowledged. It is not just about the new baby fitting in with family life, it is about the transformation of family life to include this new being.

Allow this time. Make the space in your life. Ask for help.

Stay in bed and breastfeed, caress and stroke and smell and talk to your child and allow yourself to be cared for. Sleep when your baby sleeps. Don't start doing or organizing things as soon as your baby dozes off. She needs you to be rested. Be truly responsible.

Giving birth also gives birth to the new you, the mother, and not only the mother of your child, but of all children. When you become the mother of your child, you take on something of the principle of Mother. You cannot look at other children or the suffering of others with the same eyes as before. You have been elevated to Mother.

Could it be that post-natal depression is related to a lack of support and acknowledgment of the amazing feat the mother has performed, and is continuing to perform, the absence of recognition of the tremendous value of her role as Mother?

It is as if we pretend that motherhood doesn't exist other than in the physical chores associated with caring for a baby. The spiritual side and the transformation into motherhood is not acknowledged and this leaves the mother with a sense of loss and of mourning, even though she may not be aware of what she is mourning.

It is the mourning for her birthright: conscious motherhood. Knowing what is truly important and what is not. We live in a world of topsy-turvy values. The mother's employment is seen as more important than her spiritual birth as a mother. We live our lives as if spiritual motherhood does not exist, like we pretend that death does not exist.

The Madonna and Child

The image of the Virgin and Child is a rich and potent symbol with many layers of meaning. At one level, it illustrates a principle, embodies a metaphor, represents an aim. It shows what it is possible for a woman to attain through motherhood — the sacred processes of motherhood. The suckling of the Christ child represents the building of emotional function. Woman is shown to radiate divine emanations after reaching the higher level of being by delving into the mysteries of birth and returning to nourish her child at more than merely the physical level.

It is not only the child that comes trailing clouds of glory, so too does the mother, from her journey to the real world, beyond time, beyond matter, and this is what religious imagery can show. The sacred life force flowing through matter, Mother.

Mourning period and post-natal depression

After birth a period of mourning similar to the period of lying-in is also necessary. You may be mourning for conscious motherhood, but you are also mourning for the loss of yourself: your carefree, irresponsible self. This is not the same as regret. It is part of the growing process required to become a mother, and is quite natural and should be embraced. It is also sometimes referred to as post-natal depression. If you become more seriously depressed you should of course contact your doctor. However, it is good to be aware that this is a natural phenomenon and is to be expected.

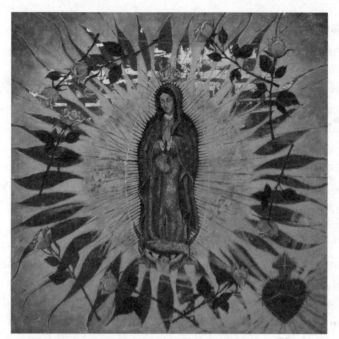

The Virgin, the birth canal and the fertilized ovum

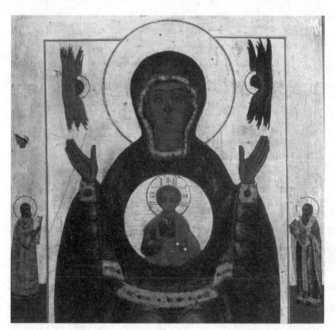

The Virgin of the Sign

The traditional period of confinement of forty days is just the beginning of the recovery, and we do not even allow that. Women who give birth in hospital are often expected to leave within 24 hours of giving birth. It is naïve to think that, educated as we are by the media and society at large, a mother will do anything but try to get back to her normal life straight away. She will be trying to tidy up, cook or interact with her other children as soon as she can get up.

Forty days was applied for good reason. It is not just your physical body that has experienced the change. Your psyche has been irrevocably re-arranged. And you are holding a small and very demanding child who requires constant attention in your arms.

This 'mourning period' can be seen as a period for the psyche to recover after the momentous events and experience of childbirth. Although it may take as little as six to eight weeks for you to recover physically, the readjustment of your psyche takes longer. I found that after each birth it took me about six months to adjust to the new order of things and to regain my balance psychologically. Of course, this depends on the individual; the important thing is that you take it into account and allow for this process to take place. Do not rush to get back to how things were before, because things cannot get back to how they were before. You and the world are irrevocably changed by the birth of this new human being.

There is a Muslim saying that states: a baby needs nine months to adjust to life in the womb and nine months to adjust to life outside the womb. Perhaps the same period applies to the mother.

Cot death

For the first few months of independent life, is it still possible to come and go, to enter and exit the physical body? This possibility diminishes as the child gradually becomes hypnotized by the world of three dimensions and her parents' responses to it. What we call cot death is perhaps when the essence of a being decides to leave even after it has fully materialized, even after it has fully entered the body by drawing its first breath. Your child has the choice to come and the choice to go.

After a certain point, she begins to forget and becomes more and more enthralled by the world of matter that fills her through our senses, just like we have been.

Bringing your womb back to preparedness

It takes about six to eight weeks for the area in your womb where your placenta was attached to heal. During this period, you will experience a bloody discharge known as lochia. The bleeding resembles your usual period for a week or so, and then gradually reduces over the next few weeks. It also takes about six to eight weeks for your uterus to return to its normal size.

One of the many benefits of breastfeeding will be felt as soon as your baby's sucking triggers the first milk ejection reflex. The pleasantly surging tension through your breast will be accompanied by a warm, gentle contraction of your womb, a bit like a period pain. Each time you breastfeed, your womb takes a step further towards regaining its original shape and size, in preparation for its next series of unfoldings. Your birth cannot be said to be fully completed until your womb is back to its normal state of preparedness. This usually takes about eight weeks.

So, when it is not hyperintended into a few hours or days, the full experience of birth may span eighteen weeks.

Breastfeeding

Biologically, breastfeeding can be described as follows: the baby suckles the breast, which stimulates the nipple receptors. These nipple receptors transmit a neurological signal to the brain. The signal triggers the release of oxytocin. The oxytocin is carried in the bloodstream and, when it reaches the breast, triggers the milk-ejection reflex. If your baby suckles for longer, more oxytocin is released. Higher levels of oxytocin in the blood increase the milk-ejection reflex. This means that your baby controls exactly how much milk is produced. In addition, the pituitary gland produces prolactin, a hormone primarily associated with lactation, which further stimulates milk production.

If your baby is still hungry after a feed, she will continue to suckle, creating more milk for herself. When your baby sucks less because she is older and eating ordinary food, less oxytocin is produced and so the milk-ejection reflex lessens. This means that you *cannot* have too little milk for your baby. You are a self-regulating organism at instinctive level.

If you let your baby suckle as much as she wants you will produce exactly as much milk as she needs. Your body is such a carefully calibrated and wondrous machine that it produces just as much milk as she is sucking for. Trust your body; it is far more intelligent than you, or your ordinary intellect, anyway. Don't try to lose weight — you will steal resources from yourself and from your baby to nourish your vanity. Leave any weight loss for later. It will happen naturally anyway unless you comfort eat, which is another issue.

It is an ecstatic experience to be able to satisfy this complete, enchanting new person's needs by placing them at your breast, to soothe their crying with your warm bosom. It is a very great privilege to be allowed to act out the role of Mother in this eternal relationship between human beings.

Breast milk is far superior to anything else you can feed your baby: it is possibly the most nutritious substance on earth. Breast milk contains specific antibodies against respiratory and intestinal bacteria and viruses. These are thought to increase a child's resistance to infection. Many studies comparing the frequency of illness between breast- and formula-fed infants demonstrate fewer and less severe illnesses in breast-fed infants. Breastfeeding has also recently been linked to a reduced risk of developing allergies and asthma. Human breast milk also contains substances that have a calming effect on newborns; breast-fed babies tend to cry less and are calmer than bottle-fed babies.

Breast milk has been termed 'environmentally-specific milk.' This means that the mother produces precisely what her newborn needs to be protected against. The mother manufactures breast milk that is tailor-made to fight precisely those organisms that the baby is most likely to be exposed to. Breast milk is a dynamic fluid that constantly changes in composition and responds to the baby's changing needs. It also provides the specific nutrients that are needed at each age and in each situation.

Breast milk simply cannot be replicated by formula, which will always be a poor substitute — and you need to know this. Pretending that it is just as good and that it doesn't really matter if you don't breastfeed your baby is doing your baby a disservice.

If, for some valid reason, you really cannot breastfeed, then so be it. That is the situation that you need to transform and to find the real, positive reason for why it had to be so. There will be one, if you open yourself to it. It may be that this will give you and your baby something that could not be had in any other way. If this is your fate, then you have the possibility of actively entering into it and of working on not getting caught up in negativity towards yourself or other women who can breastfeed. But first of all, the possibility of breastfeeding must have been exhausted.

For the first few days after birth, your breasts produce a yellow, thick liquid known as colostrum. This superb substance, which cannot be produced artificially, is full of antibodies that attach to the mucus membranes in your baby's nose, mouth, throat and stomach. Colostrum also contains enzymes that aid digestion and proteins that regulate iron.

After three or four days, your breasts will start the production of mature milk. Transitional milk is then produced for about two weeks, when immune-boosting properties gradually decrease and are replaced by fat and milk sugars. Fully mature milk is sweet and rich, although the colour varies from yellow-white to green-blue. It may be disconcerting to see your milk look thin and bluish, but this is normal. It is the richest, creamiest, sweetest, most nutritious bluish milk on earth.

Each feed provides your baby with two different kinds of milk, the foremilk and the hindmilk. The foremilk, which comes first as its name suggests, is plentiful and not so fatty and quenches your baby's thirst. The hindmilk, which comes towards the end of the feed, is more fatty and less plentiful. If you let your baby feed as often and for as long as she likes, you will ensure that she receives sufficient quantities to fill her up and the necessary fat content for healthy development.

There is a direct connection between the breasts and the uterus, perhaps a connection for the building and maintenance of emotional function. When the baby latches on to your nipple you will soon experience the milk-ejection reflex or 'let-down,' a pressure down all the multitude of ducts that comprise your breast tissue. It is a warm, urgent, pressing sensation coupled with an intense longing to be near your child. The cry of another child can sometimes trigger it, or even seeing a picture of your child. Soon after this reflex you will feel your womb contract, pulling itself together back into the perfect pear shape of holy receiving: ready, empty, clean, restored, perfect, new for the next potential child to come into the world.

Problems with breastfeeding

Most women who stop breastfeeding earlier than they would have liked to give one of the following reasons:

'I didn't have enough milk.'
As we have seen, this is simply not true. You do have enough milk. What then is the real reason? A feeling of self-doubt, a lack of confidence in your ability to breastfeed? It *is* difficult. Surprisingly difficult for something that is essential to survival.

Acknowledging that breastfeeding is not easy at first, that it requires determination, encouragement from those around you and help from more experienced women and midwives, will help. It is not a test; every woman who has given birth has faced the same difficulty and, unless she has been lucky enough to be surrounded by supportive, experienced women, the same doubts about her own ability.

'I couldn't get my baby to latch on.'
Three or four days after birth, your breasts will start the production of mature milk. You may find that as this happens, your breasts swell up and become rock hard overnight. This is usually referred to as the milk 'coming in.' Your breasts can become engorged as a result of the intense hormonal activity going on in your body, and it can be very difficult to breastfeed. To ease this, you will need to extract a little milk with your hands or a breast pump before breastfeeding, to make it easier for your

baby to latch on. There are many simple-to-use, hand-powered pumps available. Your breasts will become less full after a few days, and later they will be able to contain three times as much milk without ever needing to become so enlarged again.

It is also difficult for the child. You may see the baby struggling to take the nipple, trying desperately to latch on but not really being sure how to do it. Breastfeeding is a mutual learning process, and it is not one for which you can get a diploma beforehand. It is a shared learning experience, and overcoming this initial difficulty together brings you closer to your child. It is not just about sticking the nipple in the baby's mouth. It requires courage, determination and strength to breastfeed. Pretending that it is the easiest and most natural (meaning, here, that it ought just to happen by itself) thing in the world will only make women feel inadequate when they are confronted with the inevitable difficulties.

'My nipples were too sore to breastfeed.'
They do get very sore, but it passes. For the first few days it may be all right, but then the child may be sucking for so long and so frequently that the nipples start to crack and bleed. This is commonplace and part of the process of your nipples becoming accustomed to your child (assuming your baby is latched on correctly; poor position at the nipple can cause considerable and unnecessary damage). Fortunately, they soon become more thick-skinned. After a week or two, they will be as tough as old boots.

One way of getting through this period may be to stay away from creams and rubber caps or whatever is foist upon you from the outside, and to stick with the most healing, nourishing substance in the world: breast milk itself. Express a drop or two and rub it into your sore nipples. If you tape empty limpet shells full of breast milk onto the nipples with masking tape, the milk will soothe and bathe the nipple until the next feed. This aids fast healing, keeps the nipples supple and prevents the skin from cracking.

This may sound ridiculous, but it works, as many women will testify. It may make you face the question: how much do I actually want to breastfeed? Is avoiding appearing ridiculous for a week more important to you than breastfeeding your child? Don't be a victim of circumstance. It may be that your vanity is more important. If it is so, acknowledge it and go into the world of bottle-feeding knowingly. There is no judgment implied in this. The important thing is to know yourself and to not allow yourself to be pushed into a series of events that leave you a victim.

The most obvious benefit of breastfeeding, apart from the delectable pleasure, is that your breasts are always with you. Furthermore, the milk is always the right temperature and sterile. You always have a dummy on hand to quieten or comfort your child. At night, you don't need to get out of bed to feed your baby. You don't need to prepare, clean, disinfect, buy or throw away anything. Breastfeeding makes your life easier.

If breasts become achy and heavy, shower in warm water, massaging and stroking your breasts towards the nipple to ease any congestion. Keep your breasts warm, with wool pads tucked into your bra and warm clothing. Nurturing your breasts shows responsible behaviour towards your child, maintaining this miraculous source of love and superior nourishment. You may find that you become more aware of the full extent of your breast tissue, that it reaches well beyond what we usually call our breasts. You may experience a more ready feeling of cold on your back, shoulders and ribs.

Successful breastfeeding requires a relaxed environment and is therefore probably best begun outside of a hospital environment. If a woman is tense, it will be more difficult for her milk to begin to flow. Her baby will pick up on the tension and begin to cry, and soon a vicious circle begins. If you do give birth in hospital, capitalize on the midwives' expertise and ask them to show you the techniques. Remember that it is not easy, so don't be afraid to ask for help.

And persevere, persevere, persevere. Remember that breastfeeding is designed to work. Your body wants it to work. Your baby wants it to work. If you get through the first couple of weeks you will have at your disposal a supremely practical and beneficial source of nourishment and comfort for years to come. Breastfeeding is a way of giving love. Work to become able to give your love, through the divine nectar that flows through your physical presence.

Practical considerations during breastfeeding

It is important to remember to drink at least twice as much as usual. All that liquid drunk by the baby needs to be replaced, or you will find yourself exhausted and with a headache. So keep yourself topped up during the day, and remember to keep a bottle of water by your bedside at night.

Make sure that you arrange your clothing so that you feel comfortable breastfeeding in public. You will feel discouraged to breastfeed if you are worried about exposing too much of your ample bosoms. Many high-street clothes stores offer maternity ranges that include tops and dresses with an overlapping slit across the chest that allows you to get your breast out comfortably while avoiding exposing any flesh. This means that you can breastfeed with ease. The double layer of cloth also helps to keep your breasts warm. The 'boob' brand of breastfeeding clothes is good and to be recommended. Successful breastfeeding requires effort and forethought, and feeling comfortable about doing it anywhere you might find yourself is paramount to success.

Be proud of what you are doing. You are building a physically and emotionally healthy person, someone whose contribution to the world of tomorrow will be partly determined by how she is treated and nourished in childhood. You know that breast milk has supreme properties and provides a form of nourishment that cannot be bought. Treasure it; value it. Treat yourself with the respect you deserve as the generator of this miraculous fluid.

Sleeping together

If you sleep together, you can breastfeed without getting up, making for a calmer environment for everyone in the family, including yourself. Many women from indigenous cultures follow the child's rhythm, sleeping together at night and napping with their child during the day. It is worth noting that it is still common practice for mothers to sleep with their children in some highly industrialized nations, such as Japan.

There is no evidence to suggest an increased mortality rate because of sleeping with your child. You are extremely unlikely to roll onto your child unless you've taken drugs or are drunk.

If you are always in close proximity to your child, you will hear her breathing and be able to monitor her in a way that no electronic monitor, video link or even medical equipment ever will. You will be intuitively aware of your baby's internal functions and breathing, and be able to pick up on even the tiniest signal in the right way. Equally important, you will be able to intuitively disregard signals that a machine might pick up but which mean nothing with regard to your child's well-being.

Sleeping in the same bed as your baby stabilizes a baby's heart rate and reduces crying. It also encourages frequent breastfeeding and may reduce the risk of cot death. Most cot deaths occur when the baby is sleeping in a different room from the mother, a statistical fact that currently remains unexplained.

If the mother is right there, skin on skin next to the baby, the transition into living in a physical body may prove easier for the new being who has just come into the world. Sleeping next to your baby means that you will naturally be more aware of her, stroking, kissing and touching her much more frequently than if you were sleeping in separate rooms. You are generously affirming her physical body and her presence here on earth.

In our society there is a strong emphasis on performance. Your child is expected to perform even at a few weeks old. 'Isn't she good?' 'What a well-behaved baby!' are phrases you may hear and which are symptomatic of this idea that we ought to be valued on the basis of performance. A child that sleeps on its own from an early age is seen as performing well.

Affirming emotional function

When you breastfeed your child, you are holding her within the radiation of your hormonal emanations and secretions, in a cloud of emotion. We do not get this close to each other for such long periods or with such frequency during adult life. This closeness, touching and holding, is important for the affirmation of emotional function in the budding threefold nature of your child.

She is sharing in your emanations. Your hormones, pheromones, sweat, scent and breath all constantly communicate to her what you are feeling. She learns the emotional register from you. This process began during the nine months in the womb, and is consolidated in the outside world during the period of breastfeeding.

We know from experimentation that a baby monkey that is deprived of its mother (or any other living being to care for him) after birth becomes severely disturbed. In these notorious experiments, the baby monkeys were given only artificial warmth and softness and were fed from a bottle not held by a person. Emotional function failed to develop fully, and when mature these monkeys exhibited pathological behaviour. Newborns have an organic need to be touched and caressed in order for healthy emotional and physical development to take place.

Warmth and gentle touch triggers the release of oxytocin, a hormone shown to induce a state of calm and relaxation, engendering a sense of well-being. This is our first emotion, as we are bathed in the oxytocin passed on to us from our mother's bloodstream, and gently touched by the sides of our mother's womb and rocked in her warmth.

Touch triggers the release of oxytocin in adults as well as babies. Oxytocin allows our blood pressure to drop and our pain threshold to increase. This, in turn, reduces cortisol levels, balancing the whole system. Oxytocin release may also be triggered by a friendly tone of voice, friendly facial expressions and personal contact, although this has yet to be scientifically proven. What we can conclude, however, is that the release of oxytocin, triggered by touch and warmth, constitutes an important element of the formation of emotional function.

Emotional function is different from instinctive-moving and intellectual functions in that there is no negative part. Emotional function has only a positive part. Faith, hope and love are what rightfully belong to us. In our civilization we have become so far removed from this that we no longer recognize the distinction between an instinctive like or dislike and true emotion. A great deal of help and affirmation from our mother is needed in order not to confuse the pain and discomfort of an injury with our *feelings*, which should always be kept clean. We need help and assistance to put our experiences in the right place. And it takes time.

> Saying the Lord's Prayer together at the end of each day is a helpful practice. This prayer has been considered the most important for nearly 2,000 years for good reason. Ponder in your heart what each word means, what its significance is to you. Study the translation. How are the words chosen? Draw your own conclusions. Details of a helpful book called *A Recapitulation of the Lord's Prayer* are given in the Resources section.

Skin on skin contact transmits physical warmth and pleasure and builds confidence. It affirms the child's presence in her physical body. Touch and cuddle and hold and caress and tickle and kiss and breathe in the smell of your baby. A deep-seated confidence that will last a lifetime, the confidence of knowing that your basic needs will be met by your mother, is established by the association of physical pleasure and comfort with feeding.

The skin is the largest organ in the body. The surface of the skin is covered in thousands of nerve receptors that, when touched, trigger the release of oxytocin. Any mother knows that her loving touch soothes a crying baby, but her touch also helps to stimulate the baby's blood flow, strengthen her immune system and improve her digestion. Every time you touch your baby, supporting her in all these ways, you are also making the connection between you and her stronger and deeper.

Affirm and re-affirm her sensation of well-being in her body. She is manifest, through the delight of sensation. Affirm sensation, affirm her presence in the physical body. Affirm the wonder that she and you are alive, are here, in this moment, now.

Responding to your baby's needs

Your child cries to tell you that something is wrong. Respond to her cries and she will soon stop. The practice in hospitals of separating the mother and baby at birth can be viewed as teaching babies to cry. Studies have found that problems with colic and intensive crying appear to be largely cultural. It is our way of living and our inner states that are reflected back to us in our crying babies.

Stressed mothers often have crying babies and crying babies lead to stressed mothers. You will need a network of support around you. Prepare. Exercise forethought, and if you don't have help, ask for it. Keep asking.

Carry your baby close and respond to her needs and your baby will feel safe, secure and confident. These feelings and attitudes will permeate your baby's life right through to adulthood. It is only for a short time that your baby will make these intensive demands on you. Allow yourself to be a mother and do not try to be simultaneously a yummy mummy or an executive, and you have the possibility of giving yourself and your child long-term benefits.

Hormonal changes

The hormonal changes that you have experienced during pregnancy and childbirth continue during the period of breastfeeding. Oxytocin is known to reduce memory function, and it is thought that this might help new mothers to forget the pain of childbirth. It is possible to observe in yourself the non-intellectual and emotional state of a nursing mother.

> When my friend Pia became a mother for the first time she went out to run an errand in her car. As she approached a roundabout she noticed to her astonishment that everyone was driving around it the wrong way. She then proceeded to go round the roundabout the right way, to show all these terrible drivers how it should be done. You can image the chaos. Fortunately no one was injured, apart from a small dent in Pia's pride.

Remember to take this time fully, to set this time aside as dedicated to breastfeeding. Don't squeeze other things in. Prioritize your primary role as Mother. Your mind is instinctively focused on your child and so it should be. You are the keeper of your tissues. Maintain and nourish yourself well so that you may maintain and nourish well. Supplement your diet with vitamins and try to eat fresh, organic and healthy food.

Milk teeth

Perhaps breastfeeding is intended by nature to continue until the milk teeth are expelled, hence the name 'milk teeth.' These teeth are expendable and can be used during the transitional stage between breast milk and solid food. Breast milk is very sweet and causes teeth to rot, so if our adult teeth erupted at six months many of them would be destroyed by the time we got to seven.

We do not breastfeed for nearly long enough in our civilization. How old is the Christ child being breastfed in some paintings? Although prolonged breastfeeding is certainly not the only reason why his depicted age is greater than we might consider appropriate today, this is a consideration.

Breastfeeding may take the full seven years assigned to her in the child's development, including the gradual transition to solid food. This is not to say that we should all flout convention in a civilization far removed from what is natural and right, from what is truly normal. However, if we can become aware of it, it may help to put things into perspective. Breastfeeding is as important as pregnancy and birth in the development of emotional function.

An extended period of breastfeeding also serves as a natural means of birth control, as your fertility is significantly reduced during this time.

11. Motherhood

Your child in the world

It has been said that the first seven years of a child's life belong to the mother. Expressed in terms of a triad, comprising the principles of active, passive and neutralizing, the mother acts as the active principle for this period. She cares for and protects the baby, who is passive. During this period, the father embodies the neutralizing principle. The next seven years have been said to belong to the father. The child is bigger, exploring the world around him and living more under her father's guidance. The father is then active while the child remains passive. During this period, the mother embodies the neutralizing principle. The third seven-year period has been said to belong to culture, to society, to the child's peers. The peers are active, the child remains passive and her parents are neutralizing.

When the child reaches the age of 21, a triad on a larger scale becomes manifest: 3 x 7 = 21. At 21, he reaches the age of responsibility and his life becomes fully his own. Here he embodies the active principle for the first time. This is when his real education should begin, but where our civilization allows it to stop. This is when he is ready to begin to think about the meaning of existence and why we are here. What role have I come here to play, now that I am an adult?

In the Christian church, we find ritual markers indicating the importance of these seven-year intervals: baptism, first holy communion, confirmation, marriage.

This information may be of use if it helps you to stop fighting the natural developmental phases associated with growing up. Of course, it does not mean that you, the mother, wash your hands of your child from the age of seven! But it may be helpful to consider this when raising your child. And it may help to allow your partner to play their part fully.

But the newborn, with his sweet-smelling breath and soft, downy hair, deep all-knowing gaze and urgent lips and hands, belongs to his mother. You have shared the same blood, the same hormonal secretions, experienced the same biochemical changes and lived in the same emotions for nine months. On one level, the instinctive, this makes you closer than you can ever hope to be to your partner. But you were once this close to your own mother. That is why she is so important to you, still.

The blood connection

You and your baby have had a literal blood connection for nine months, and have developed finely attuned paths of communication. This continues for a time outside the womb, perhaps even for a few years. When your child cries, you can sometimes hear from the cry what part of her anatomy is hurt and how serious the incident.

Listen to this inner voice, with your inner ear, and keep seeing with your inner eye what the child sees with hers. These faculties are not acknowledged by our civilization and so receive no stimulus during those crucial early months and years. If your child's experience is never affirmed or acknowledged, it gradually becomes less and less real. The child imitates you and your responses. If he gets no confirmation of that silent communication, he will stop regarding his experiences as anything worthwhile.

We have seen that if a kitten's eyes are taped over at birth, and the tape removed at ten weeks, the cat will never be able to see. If a function is never validated, it will atrophy. Why are our brains so large? Why do we use such a tiny proportion of our real brain capacity? What is it that we have lost sight of in this civilization?

Help your child according to your own abilities, acknowledge shared experiences and give a name to your child's ability to see what is not immediately before his eyes. But remain wary of fuelling imagination — this is a tightrope walk. Stop this practice as soon as you sense that you or your child is crossing over into make-believe or fantasy.

Speaking

He is like a sponge, eager and keen to engage with you and to learn from you. If you clearly mouth and say words to him, he will soon begin to imitate you. At first only the lip movements, but if you persist the sounds too will come. It is possible to hear your baby try to say 'hello' (ero) after only a few weeks. In itself, this copying of words might not mean much, but it shows how incredibly willing and with what a forceful dynamic for learning we come into the world. Your newborn child's enthusiasm for life is boundless. And it is you that he wishes, with all his being, to copy.

Motherhood

One of the reasons often cited for going back to work soon after having a child is, 'I needed to have a life.' The implication is that being a mother, taking care of your own children, is not really having a life. Are we so abnormal as women today that we are unable to rightly value nature's main purpose for our existence, our primary life duty? The most sacred duty in a woman's life is motherhood. The abnormality is compounded by the low status assigned to being a stay-at-home mum. Profession, spending-power and appearance are the most highly-valued attributes in our society. The consequence is that women who try to live more normally, to strive to fulfil their highest potential as mothers, feel unacknowledged. There is no recognition of the gargantuan effort they are making.

To begin with, it may be enough that your partner recognizes it, but in the long run it can wear you down. You need to remain on your guard. It is our civilization whose values are upside down, not your choice to look after your own children. Watch, and be ready; the time will soon come when your children are all at school and you will have more time to yourself.

Real Possibilities

Theodor's birth

About a month before he was born my womb appeared to me in a reverie. I wasn't asleep in the way you are at night but lying resting, dreaming. My womb appeared to my consciousness, no physical form, just a presence that stated, expressed, radiated, not spoken with words, that everything was going to be fine and that he was taking over now. It felt masculine, like a general or colonel, very authoritative and self-assured. As soon as I became aware of this strange image and experience I quickly tried to ask what I was supposed to do in all this that he seemed to know so much about, but he was gone before I could even register the thought. This happened in a microsecond, in a flash. It was so quick.

He came carefully, considerately. Contractions started around midday. I had lunch, which I promptly threw up. First timer's nerves. I worked steadily in my mother's living room, staring at the globe as each contraction passed through me. Antananarivo is the capital of Madagascar. It is indelibly etched into my consciousness.

As the contractions speeded up we decided to go to the hospital. I managed to get down the stairs with difficulty. The car didn't start. We had to change cars. I was nervous. We travelled to hospital. Every time the car went over a bump it hurt much more.

I got to hospital and after about half an hour of procedures I was in a room and could start working again. It took a while for contractions to build up again. I was examined. When I felt the momentum coming hard and fast and had turned back into my world of work, the midwife told me her shift was finished. This was devastating. It was as if God would tell you his shift was finished and that the world had to end right now.

'Unfortunately that's just the way it is.' I was gutted. There was no self-pity, just impossibility. The new midwife came, introduced herself. Another half hour of messing around, disturbance. She sat down in a corner and looked at her stopwatch. This made me nervous and uncomfortable. The contractions slowed down. I felt tense and the midwife didn't speak to me and I didn't speak to her. Contractions slowed further. I decided I had to take responsibility for my situation and I asked her to leave and to get another midwife.

This is something I am immensely proud of. It was difficult. I was vulnerable and it would have been so much easier to go with the flow and not be a nuisance. She was hurt and hesitant about going at first, but she went.

The new midwife came. It took about half an hour to get going again. She was matronly and radiated the calm confidence that vast experience brings. She told me to get angry, to think of all the swearwords I knew and utter them at the next contraction. I did and out he popped, literally popped, like a champagne cork cum slippery seal.

He slid over my clitoris and intense pleasure pulsed through my loins. Pleasure very close to pain. My husband caught him and danced and levitated with joy. He shone.

I was not back in my body yet. This was not disconcerting: my state was already so much out of the ordinary. I just observed that I could not sense my body. The baby was placed on my chest and I felt no sensation in my fingers and arms or my chest. It took about ten minutes for me to return.

During these ten minutes the child gazed intently into my eyes and told me all the mysteries he had just seen. He knew who I was, why he had come and what he had to do. He recognized me. His incredible intensity and energy helped me to recognize him. As we gazed star-struck into each other's eyes sensation slowly returned to my fingers and I realized I was nestling a little testicle in my left hand. Tears welled up in my eyes. It was a boy!

The midwife clocked the time. It was twenty past midnight. Twenty minutes into my husband's 31st birthday.

Theodor had moved around so vigorously in the womb that he had tied his umbilical cord into a knot. I still keep the knotted section of umbilical cord amongst my most treasured possessions.

The placenta was massaged out by the midwife after about forty minutes. I tore and had no stitches. There were no complications.

Breastfeeding was difficult at first. He wasn't keen until after a good few hours. The midwives in hospital offered very good and practical advice about how to get him to latch on. This was followed up later during home visits. Some adjustments to my breastfeeding technique were necessary. My nipples became sore and bleeding after a week and it lasted for about a week. I breastfed for three years.

Ella's birth

She named herself to me in a dream, an afternoon reverie. She appeared with the face of an older woman and simply showed herself and gave the name Ella. There was no doubt what it meant. It was so quick it was over before I could register what was happening or try to respond or even observe. I was uncertain and doubted that it was real. How can we tell the difference between what is real and imagination? I told only my husband about this.

She came quickly, like a spring flood. My mucal plug went at around three p.m. I had a big bowl of pasta and went to rest and got some sleep, maybe half an hour. I got up and went to my desk and continued typing. Contractions were coming quicker. I stood up to meet each contraction at my desk and typed in between. I spoke to my husband as we were working together.

At about six I went downstairs and worked, standing, moving around: hanging on the benches in the sauna, leaning on my husband, kneeling on the sofa. I got in the warm water of the birthing pool when the pain became hard to meet. I was swept away in the comfort and lightness of the supporting water. I calmed.

It was early spring in Sweden, mid-April, and snow was still on the ground outside the window. I saw the first green shoots pushing up through the snow and the buds of white wood anemones nodding in the cold breeze. They are her flowers; Easter is her time. She kept on coming. Just before she pushed through the final barrier I screamed in agony of death, full of fear for a moment. I screamed without holding back.

Then she came. I was urged by the midwife to reach out for her, put my hands down to receive her. I said I couldn't. She reassured me and said that of course I could. So I did and I received my own child from my womb. I took her with my own hands, from my own womb. It was ecstasy. Everyone was laughing, crying, smiling. She had come.

It was Easter Monday.

I gazed into her eyes looking for recognition, as I had come to expect this from my previous experience with Theodor. That is not what she is about. She started to look around her straight away. She knew where she was and why she had come and what she had to do and she set about it with vigour. As I felt the absence of testicles I was stunned. It *was* Ella, Ella who had named herself, who had come.

I tore and had no stitches. I have a scar from this of which I am enormously proud.

The placenta came soon afterwards of its own accord. I pulled very gently on the umbilical cord to help it out.

I thought breastfeeding was going to be easy now that I was so experienced. But my breasts were hard as coconuts and she couldn't latch on. I had to struggle and keep trying and sweating and hurting for a few days. I had sore nipples for about a week. Mastitis threatened a few times and was resolved with massage and hot showers and plenty of sucking. I breastfed for two years.

Gabriel's birth

I dreamed that he was Gabriel. He appeared to me as a baby. I didn't like this name at all when I woke up. I ignored the dream and talked about naming him Leonard, Caedmon, Michael.

I was out with Ella and Theodor a few days before the birth when I was suddenly overcome by strong contractions. I went into a car repair workshop nearby and sat down on a stool while the contractions passed through me. After a while they subsided and I stood up to go home. I looked down on the stool I had been sitting on to check my waters hadn't broken, and the name Gabriel was emblazoned on it. Now that was a shock.

I went outside with Ella and Theodor and as we got into the car to drive home, I saw in the window of the car repair workshop a large poster saying, 'Give Life,' spoken by a mechanical android. Now I knew. The choice was not mine. He was Gabriel. I went back after the birth to take photos of the stool and the poster.

Gabriel came quietly in the night. The mucal plug had gone a week before, prompting everyone into a frenzy of anticipation. Day after day of small contractions followed. I had been visualizing my uterus opening, unfurling, since week 38 and I think this was happening still. A slow, gentle birth.

The final phase came softly, calmly, forcefully, like velvet in the night. I awoke at about midnight to contractions. I went downstairs and lent into large pillows I had prepared. I disappeared into the spiral whirlwind of descent into the mysteries beyond time. I fell and fell, deeper and deeper, into the well of life.

In the dark I worked quietly. Still, peaceful and calm. Contractions intensified. There was no fear. Just deep, still confidence. I called Adam but he thought it would be hours before he needed to come down. It was three o'clock in the morning. At half past three I got into the water as it was feeling very strong and painful. The water soothed me a little but not as much as with Ella. The power just kept on increasing and rushing through me and it was unbearably painful.

Adam came down as I was lowing loudly by now. He called the midwife. She came quickly and asked to examine me, which I forcefully declined as I was about to exit my body by way of the pores. A fox passed silently directly outside the window through which I was staring into the distance. The fox was about twenty centimetres away from me, woman, giving birth. I saw every blade of grass, every dewdrop in the rising sun in such an intensely real way. I have that image etched in my mind forever.

I felt him crowning and reached down to touch his golden head. I held back during one contraction, as I was now experienced enough to be able to do this. I felt his hard head and let him slip through my moist tissues and into my arms. His umbilical cord was tangled round his neck and with balletic dexterity and unintrusiveness the midwife removed it as if it were the simplest and most natural thing in the world, which it was.

I took him into my arms but couldn't quite lift him to my chest as the umbilical cord was tangled round my leg. This required some manoeuvring with the help of the midwife and Adam, and I eventually held him close to my chest. He was so calm and present, so steady. So secure that this was right. He had come to the right place, carefully chosen by him. We greeted him. It was 4.44 in the morning.

Adam went upstairs and made a big bacon and egg breakfast which all three of us devoured. We called my mother and she arrived in a taxi with Ella and Theodor by six o'clock.

I did not tear. I squatted to push out the placenta by myself. Of this, too, I am immensely proud. I was active. Nothing was *done* to me. I did it.

Breastfeeding was smooth, as the experience with Ella had shown me not to overestimate my expertise or underestimate the uniqueness of each child's sucking. Gabriel went straight for the breast as soon as he was out. I used limpets filled with breast milk taped to my breasts to ease sore nipples. I breastfed Gabriel for a year and a half.

Resources

This is a personal selection of books and other resources that I have found useful for developing my approach. It is in no way exhaustive or authoritative. You are the foremost expert on what you need!

Books

Birth Reborn: What Childbirth Should Be, Michel Odent, Souvenir Press Ltd, London, 1994.
— Michel Odent has been instrumental in influencing the history of childbirth and health research for decades. He introduced the concept of birthing pools and stressed the importance of a home-like environment during childbirth. Michel Odent developed a maternity unit in France where he oversaw one thousand births a year while maintaining ideal statistics and very low rates of intervention and later went on to work through home birth. He is the author of fifty scientific papers and eleven books.

Homebirth and Other Alternatives to Hospital, Sheila Kitzinger, Dorling Kindersley, London, 1991.
— An essential guide for any woman wanting to make an informed choice about her birthing experience. Wonderful photographs and birth stories.

Ina May's Guide to Childbirth, Ina May Gaskin, Vermillion, London, 2008.
— Ina May Gaskin founded the Farm Midwifery Centre in the US and uses an intuitive approach to assist the natural birthing process. The Farm is well known for its low rates of intervention and safe statistics. She lectures all over the world, teaches midwifery, writes books and articles and edits her quarterly journal, *The Birth Gazette*. She is also the author of *Spiritual Midwifery*.

New Active Birth: A Concise Guide to Natural Childbirth, Janet Balaskas, Thorsons, London, 1990.
— Janet Balaskas is the founder of the Active Birth Movement, aimed at encouraging women to walk, stand, squat, lie and move their bodies freely during labour and birth.

A Child is Born, Lennart Nilsson, Doubleday, London, 2004.
— A classic photographic record of the journey from the egg and sperm all the way through to birth. It was first published in 1965 and is regularly updated using the latest technology to reveal close-ups of the miracle of human reproduction and the growing foetus. It also provides information on new discoveries in genetics, environmental factors, fertility treatment and pregnancy health.

Childbirth and Authoritative Knowledge: Cross-Cultural Perspectives, ed. R. E. Davis-Floyd & C. F. Sargent, University of California Press, 1997.
— Gives a good background to our unspoken assumptions about childbirth in the West and provides an insight into childbirth in a number of different cultures.

Serpent in the Sky: The High Wisdom of Ancient Egypt, John Anthony West, Quest Books, Illinois, 1996.
— This fascinating book provides access to the remarkable work of Schwaller de Lubicz on ancient Egyptian technology, symbolism, psychological training and wisdom.

The Opening of the Way: A Practical Guide to the Wisdom Teachings of Ancient Egypt, Isha Schwaller de Lubicz, Inner Traditions, Vermont, 1981.
— Written by the wife of Schwaller de Lubicz, this helpful and practical book provides access to 'difficult' and complex ideas about inner psychological transformation. Based on the Hermetic teachings of ancient Egypt, so close to the source of all esoteric traditions.

The Little Prince, Antoine de Saint-Exupéry, Egmont, London, 1991.
— A simple and effective description of mental housekeeping that speaks directly to the subconscious mind, which should rightfully be our conscious mind. Also good for reading to your child!

Mother of God, Lawrence Cunningham, Harper & Row, New York, 1982.
— A lovely selection of images of the Virgin and child from around the world.

In Search of the Miraculous: Fragments of an Unknown Teaching, P.D. Ouspensky, Arkana, New York, 1988.
— This remarkable book describes the esoteric teaching of G.I. Gurdjieff in the early years in Russia

A Beginner's Guide to Constructing the Universe, Michael S. Schneider, Avon Books, New York, 2003.
— A wonderful exploration of the deeper meanings of number and how to understand and use sacred geometry.

The Western Esoteric Traditions: A Historical Introduction, N. Goodrick-Clarke, Oxford University Press, 2008.
— A scholarly introduction to the history of the major esoteric teachings of the western world.

The Underlying Religion: An Introduction to the Perennial Philosophy, Eds. Martin Lings & Clinton Minnaar, World Wisdom, Indiana, 2007.
— An anthology of essays by leading thinkers in esoteric or

comparative religious thought, associated with René Guénon, Ananda Coomaraswamy, and Frithjof Schuon. The book addresses the fundamental truth that lies at the heart of all the great religions, revealing the connections between the different paths that all lead to the same summit.

Icons and the Mystical Origins of Christianity, Richard Temple, Element
    Books, London, 1990.
— A wonderful exposition of how to read icons and understand what they contain, opening up a world of deep symbolism.

A Recapitulation of the Lord's Prayer, anon., Eureka Editions, Utrecht, 2000.

Beyond Belief: The Secret Gospel of Thomas, Elaine Pagels, Random
    House, New York, 2003.
— As well as containing a translation into modern English of the (short) Gospel of Thomas, Elaine Pagels traces the early history of Christianity, describing how it developed from its esoteric roots into the established church of the Empire of the Roman Papacy.

On Love, A.R. Orage, The Unicorn Press, New York, 1932.

The Oragean Version, C. Daly King, privately printed in a limited
    edition of 100 copies, New York, 1951.

Online resources

www.homebirth.org.uk
A useful starting point for research.

www.jeyarani.com
Dr Gowri Motha's Gentle Birth Method aims to prepare a woman for birth through methods including self-hypnosis. Having worked as an obstetrician in a hospital setting, which she ultimately found unsatisfactory in terms of women's birth experiences, she began

investigating the alternative methods of her native Sri Lanka and South India and went on to develop her own birthing method. The self-hypnosis CDs are excellent and resonate with the holistic approach to childbirth expressed in this book.

www.hypnobirthing.com
Another self-hypnosis method with practitioners around the world.

www.joyousbirth.info
Australian website containing useful information and a young perspective.

www.llli.org
La Leche League International is a worldwide network aiming to help mothers to breastfeed by supporting each other and giving advice, encouragement, and information. It aims to increase the understanding of the importance of breastfeeding for healthy development.

www.templegallery.com
This specialist icon gallery has a wonderful collection of deeply spiritual images, some of them particularly suited to meditation for mothers and mothers-to-be. Dick Temple, who runs it, is one of the world's foremost experts on icons and a treasure trove of knowledge and understanding of the symbology behind icons.

www.gurdjieff-internet.com
Website with articles, interviews and other resources relating to esoteric teaching today.

A Guide to Child Health

Michaela Glöckler, Wolfgang Goebel

This acclaimed guide to children's physical, psychological and spiritual development is now available in a revised edition. Combining medical advice with issues of upbringing and education, this is a definitive guide for parents.

This book outlines the connection between education and healing, with all that this implies for the upbringing and good health of children. Medical, educational and religious questions often overlap, and in the search for the meaning of illness it is necessary to study the child as a whole — as body, soul and spirit.

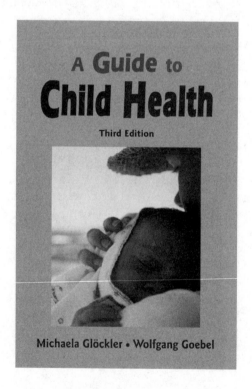

florisbooks.co.uk

Baby's First Year

Growth and Development from 0 to12 months

Paulien Bom, Machteld Huber

A baby's first year presents parents with a variety of challenges. The initial excitement of pregnancy is followed by the child's birth and subsequent development, but many parents feel in need of significant support and information regarding the more mundane areas of daily life, such as nutrition and hygiene.

This practical guide takes a holistic approach to the growth and development of a baby. Written by doctors qualified in both conventional and anthroposophical medicine, it deals with all aspects of the care of a small child up to the age of twelve months.

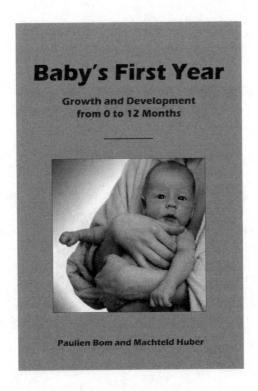

florisbooks.co.uk

Crying and Restlessness in Babies

A Parent's Guide to Natural Sleeping

Ria Blom

Every parent knows the sound of a baby who won't settle down to sleep. Crying and restlessness, especially in young babies, can be both distressing and tiring.

Ria Blom is an expert in swaddling — ways of wrapping babies securely, to help them relax naturally into sleep. Swaddling works by inducing a sense of safety and comfort in the baby — and it can work wonders for the parent as well!

This book offers quick solutions for parents under immediate stress, as well as plenty of background information about sleeping patterns and baby routines.

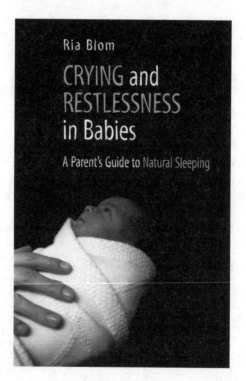

florisbooks.co.uk